BLACK CREATIVE HEALING

of related interest

Music Therapy in a Multicultural Context
A Handbook for Music Therapy Students and Professionals
Edited by Melita Belgrave and Seung-A Kim
ISBN 978 1 78592 798 0
eISBN 978 1 78450 807 4

Restorative Yoga for Ethnic and Race-Based Stress and Trauma
Gail Parker
Forewords by Octavia F. Raheem and Amy Wheeler
Illustrated by Justine Ross
ISBN 978 1 78775 185 9
eISBN 978 1 78775 186 6

Therapy in Colour
Intersectional, Anti-Racist and Intercultural Approaches by Therapists of Colour
Edited by Dr Isha Mckenzie-Mavinga, Kris Black, Karen Carberry, and Eugene Ellis
ISBN 978 1 83997 570 7
eISBN 978 1 83997 571 4

BLACK CREATIVE HEALING

Arts-based Approaches to Imagining Liberation and Addressing Race-based Trauma

Adenike Webb, PhD, MT-BC
and **Natasha Thomas,** PhD, MT-BC

Jessica Kingsley Publishers
London and Philadelphia

First published in Great Britain in 2026 by Jessica Kingsley Publishers
An imprint of John Murray Publishing Group

2

A CIP catalogue record for this title is available from the British Library and the Library of Congress

ISBN 978 1 80501 768 4
eISBN 978 1 80501 769 1

Printed and bound in the United States by Integrated Books International

Jessica Kingsley Publishers' policy is to use papers that are natural, renewable and recyclable products and made from wood grown in sustainable forests. The logging and manufacturing processes are expected to conform to the environmental regulations of the country of origin.

Jessica Kingsley Publishers
Carmelite House
50 Victoria Embankment
London EC4Y 0DZ

www.jkp.com

John Murray Publishing Group
Part of Hodder & Stoughton Ltd
An Hachette Company

The authorized representative in the EEA is Hachette Ireland,
8 Castlecourt Centre, Dublin 15, D15 XTP3, Ireland (email: info@hbgi.ie)

Contents

Acknowledgements

Who would we be without our community? *Black Creative Healing* as a book would never have existed without the interest, support, energy, and guidance of many people.

Our heartfelt appreciation goes out to the editorial and publishing staff at Jessica Kingsley Publishers for inviting us on this writing journey and guiding us along the way.

We are also grateful for the investigative and organizational efforts of our work-study student, Caroline Patterson, one of many who have helped (and continue to help!) with the administrative labor of BCH over the years.

A special shout out goes to our supporters, whether you listened to our podcast episodes, joined our online events, or became members of our Patreon or Discord spaces. Your willingness to learn, share, create, listen, laugh, rant, mourn, and dream with us have made Black Creative Healing something powerfully beautiful and dynamic.

To our parents, spouses, children, and siblings: the words, "thank you" and "we love you" don't begin to express how deeply we feel your support and have been made better by it.

And the highest respect and honor we offer to our Ancestral mothers, fathers, and kin, who not only gave us their blood, but their stories, visions, hopes, and magic. May this work we have been called to do reflect your essence and spirit and may it strengthen the bonds among all your descendants in the African Diaspora. Asé!

Acknowledgements

Invocation

There is land inside.
There are relatives beyond.
I am a tender tendon.
I sing into the fibers,
I sing into the strain,
I sing for the many that will come,
and those that remain.

NATASHA, IN AN IMPROVISED VOCAL PERFORMANCE, NATIONAL CONVENING OF THE BRITISH ASSOCIATION FOR MUSIC THERAPY, 2024

Introduction to Black Creative Healing

There is a sort of pseudo-tradition inside Afro-Caribbean families when taking an outdoor portrait of someone: there must be at least one photo of that person touching a tree.

We (Natasha and Adenike) don't know where this tradition came from, but both of us can identify in our minds countless photos of multiple family members standing amidst some form of foliage, with at least one hand on a tree. Speaking with members of other Indigenous Diasporas, we've found that there are other peoples who take pictures of family members touching plants too, and for whom this practice has become somewhat of an inside joke. These are often the pictures our people turn to when selecting images of loved ones for funeral programs, displaying them on their mantles, or in other times and places of prominence in their households. Clearly this is something that holds significance for us! But why? Why are those pictures significant to us? What are we connecting (or trying to connect) to when we put ourselves in these poses and then elevate these pictures to such places of significance in our lives? What does it all mean? And why might that meaning matter?

For me (Adenike), touching a tree, shrub (or bush, as we say in the Caribbean!), or flower reminds me that I am part of something greater than myself. The same molecules and energy that are present in me are present in it as well. As different as we are, we are alike in terms of our needs to breathe and grow. I rely on it for oxygen, food, and beauty. It relies on me for care, pruning, and nourishing. I remember that I exist in relationship to others through the carrying on of traditions or daily interactions I have, as well as in relationship to the environment around me.

Whenever I (Natasha) touch a tree, I sometimes find myself wondering what that tree has borne witness to. How many other hands it has been touched (or perhaps held!) by and for what purposes. I imagine generations of humans and other beings moving past this tree, whether they were aware of touching it or not, if for only a moment or an extended period of time, for shelter or rest, balance, or some other purpose. Then I begin to wonder about where those other humans or beings may have been going, on their way past the tree. As my mind's eye zooms out from the single tree to the garden or forest containing it, I wonder about the lives of the people on the land that is currently holding me: one generation back, two, or three. I think about how I am connected to those humans now, simply by touching something they once touched, knowing that where I feel that one point of connection, there are infinitely more points, within my own body and beyond.

Inside each human body is something like 3 billion base (chemical) pairs of DNA, 99% of which are identical between individuals.[1] Let's put this another way: inside each of us are trillions of cells, most of which are nearly identical to the over 8 billion other people on the planet.[2] The differences between us come down to interpretation and expression of those genes/cells, resulting in a kaleidoscope of skin tones, hair types, eye shapes, and differing ways of seeing/speaking/doing/being in the world.

Imagine for a moment what this means. Each of us, containing trillions of cells that link us to each other, interpreted and expressed through our Ancestors in exponential directions, each one having a unique human experience.

All our existences are woven together, across space and time, at the cellular level.

If you sit with that awareness—as in, take a moment and just read that previous sentence a few more times until your mind can see it and/or hear it without looking at the page or hearing it read aloud—what happens inside you? Physically? Emotionally? Cognitively?

For me (Natasha), I feel in myself a sort of "filling up," almost as if

I might cry, imagining the billions of us alive at this time, our strands of DNA woven together in a cloth our Ancestors are very much still a part of. I define that urge to cry as a sort of "ecstatic grief." I am ecstatic because the awesomeness of that connection holds such an almost unfathomable potential for me (and potential almost always excites me). Imagine, sharing 99% of your DNA with someone living a completely different life across the world! And I am grieving because I know my own history, and enough of others', to be aware of what horrific actions humanity has taken (and is still taking, around the world) with that potential.

For me (Adenike), I become aware of how I carry within me genetically a sense of how my long-ago Ancestors viewed their world and their place in it, their relationships to what surrounded them, sustained them, and connected them to each other. I also carry in me your Ancestors as you carry mine. I am linked at my essence to all that lives on this Earth. How can I be whole if that sustaining link is broken by fear, hate, greed, injustice? Healing becomes my intentional journey of restoration and repair—returning to a state of connection, re-membering (as in, recalling and reassembling!) myself in the legacy of humanity.

Whatever comes to your body/mind, whether it feels like a lot or not much of anything, take a breath now, and let it pass. Now take another. And another. Let yourself connect firmly to the now; to the sights and sounds around you, wherever you are, to the feeling of your clothes against your skin, the temperature of the room, and the rhythm of your own body. All these elements, co-existing together.

As you settle (back) into the "now," what does your body/mind want to do with what you've just read and/or experienced? Perhaps you just want to spend an extra moment with your breath or stretch your body in some way. Maybe you feel a need to write something down or say something aloud (to yourself or someone else); or maybe you want to do none of these things or something entirely unique to you that would make meaning out of this moment. Whatever it is, take a moment to do that now, in the space between this paragraph and the one to come, or the physical space near you. Take a moment of action, now.

This micro-cosmic experience of taking a moment to venture into a thing (an idea, a feeling, a thought), conceptualize it in whatever form your body/mind takes it, sit with it, name what emerges, and breathe your way back into a moment of action in the present is a glimpse into what we mean when we speak of Black Creative Healing.

There are some things Black folks just get about each other and the world we live in, without it having to be said. Like the thing with taking pictures of our family members touching trees. We all do it, but no one really talks about it. There can be a lot of code in a glance, a slight tilt of the head, the gentle pressure of fingertips on a shoulder, or an object of significance. Our bodies have a whole subliminal way of communicating, both within ourselves and with each other.

Many groups of people do this. And some things can be translated (or co-opted) between groups. That said, there are some non-Black folks who may pick up on a "thing" that Black folks are communicating from moment to moment. Even if they can't quite articulate what the thing is, they know something's happening. We feel it in our bodies, communicating wordlessly across all kinds of distance. And sometimes all you really need is for two people, Black or otherwise, to recognize something's going down in order for that joint attention to lead to some sort of action.

A lot of us, Black and non-Black alike, realize that something's been "going down" in relation to Black bodies and minds for generations. We haven't been ok for a long time.

The effects, responses, and histories of trauma live in our bodies. In the last 20 years, several researchers have found evidence that the sensations caused by, and the reactions to, distressing and devastating experiences that a group of people may have experienced (e.g., natural disaster, systemic oppression, war) can become encoded in us on a genetic level, such that the bodies and actions of our descendants will show signs of it several generations down the line, resulting in increased risk of things like heart disease or cancer. These are things that can literally shorten a person's lifespan. This is what we mean when we talk about intergenerational trauma;[3] [4] it is not just "bad nerves," as our grandmothers may have referred to it in generations past. It is a silent and slow taker of marginalized lives that must be faced in order to be stopped.

With this knowledge, that trauma can be handed down intergenerationally, what's to say that healing can't be too? If trauma can be encoded into our bodies in such a way that the effects can be seen generations down the line, then arguably, the potential for action—for change and for healing—also lives, has lived, and will continue to live in our bodies.

This book is for those people, Black or non-Black, who want to go from "recognizing something's going down" to making sense of and responding to "the thing" from our own bodies, and who recognize Black needs as requiring unique attention and care. This book is not for people who are looking to be saviors; this book requires that you reject the idea of being "the one" who will fix everything. Rather, it requires that you understand yourself in relation to Blackness, and Black people, and recognize that to be in true community with Black folks, our unique needs must not be pitied, flattened, or pathologized. This book is for those who understand that for all of us to get more free, one of the best things we can do for each other is to create and protect the critical space we all need for tending to ourselves and each other, including Black beings in all their wholeness and complexity, with care.

When I (Natasha) first crafted the phrase "Black Creative Healing" (affectionately shortened to BCH) as the name for a videoblog[5] and accompanying social media space[6] in 2019, I was coming from a place of general dissatisfaction with the profession of music therapy that I had been calling my professional "home" for over a decade at that point. It didn't feel like home anymore. It felt like a place where I was only accepted so long as I didn't make waves. But I'm a child of the Caribbean, "of Shipwreck and Volcano," as I often say. Sometimes all I know is waves! I wanted my work to be a place where I felt more whole and for it to have a name that honored the sociopolitical impact of my African and Caribbean Ancestors, who I want to be very clear in this moment to name as Indigenous peoples. This emphasis is important because I wanted my Ancestral and Indigenously rooted work to have a focus on well-being that was not bound to the dominant western (Eurocentric, Christian-dominant, heteronormative, sexist, and ableist) way of viewing the world. I wanted something that invited connection between my historically severed Indigenous roots—and the roots of others like me—and the roots of those Indigenous peoples who have been able to sustain their connections despite the impacts of colonization: something to recognize the similarity of our wounds while honoring the distinct differences between us. Something to serve as an identifier for a shared process, even if our points of origin and destination may differ. Thus emerged the name, as a recognition of all that we African Diasporic Peoples were, are, and could be, in community. We are Black Creative(s), healing, engaging in an ecological process of sustaining our connection to the whole: the whole that came before us, the whole that is, and the whole that is yet to come.

In this book, we hope to identify paths towards healing that are not just creative in an "innovative" sense but rooted in our own experiences as Afro-Indigenous descendants, built from years of our own creative and community-based work. We believe everyone is creative, in their own way, that creative practices have been honed generationally and culturally by our Ancestors, and that each form of creativity has a vital role to play in connection with others. There is no way we can possibly build a better world without first being able to dream it is possible, and no way a dream can be made a reality without many minds (and hands!) coming together to develop it. That, to us, is what makes this process unique and critical: it is not just "self-work." This is self-in-Ancestral-context work: creativity in community, with Africa and her children at its center.

The focus on community—all of us getting a bit more free, one relationship at a time—is part of what has spurred BCH on as a project, as well as a process. Honoring our Blackness was/is step one because it has had the most historically fraught relationship with every other aspect of our personal identities, and as relationships felt central to healing, that made it critical to prioritize the core mission objective of tending to our Black communities.

Creativity has been both our strategy and our toolbox; within every new piece of content we release, or event we hold, both the planning process and content itself has had to be creative. This has involved no small amount of flexibility, or willingness for the process (or our own ways of doing/being) to shape-shift. And all this, again, is influenced by our relationships to each other and the world we imagine to be possible.

Since the creation of the videoblog in 2019, BCH has evolved from the more passively consumable forms of media podcasting[7] to an increasingly active virtual wellness space and growing online collective, largely due to the catalyzing process of coming together as Natasha and Adenike, in mid-2020, to deepen the work together. For a time, we were simply two Black music therapists having critical conversations that we occasionally recorded, but as our conversations ignited additional relationships, we became Adenike and Natasha plus a retreat planning team, leading to the growing community of Black Creatives we regularly engage with in physical and virtual spaces today. Some of us come from the Creative Arts Therapies or other allied health spaces; others do not. Regardless of our origins, all of us are sharing our knowledge and growing together, and so is our healing capacity.

This book is organized into sections that encourage you to assess and expand your own healing capacity while reflecting on the past, present, and possibilities for the future, all while staying connected to your body in real time along the way. This is not an experience that most folks raised in dominant western culture are familiar with. We live in a world that encourages detachment from the body by prioritizing what you think over what you feel rather than encouraging the body and mind to work together. So, we will ease you into the process of exploring concepts like African Diasporic history and practices, in the context of our current global society, moving between the intellectual and the felt (embodied) senses with investigative and creative prompts that we will call, respectively, "Tap in for Reflection," and "Pour into Practice." These prompts are embedded in the chapter text and also sectioned out in a companion workbook appendix that has text boxes for journaling. Alternatively, you may wish to utilize a fresh notebook of your own for journaling your way through the prompts in those Reflection/Practice sections or for any thoughts or feelings that may emerge for you while reading through the more cognitive sections of this text. Options for exploration abound!

We encourage you to pace yourself as you move through this process. Often, when we learn things that excite or motivate us in new ways, it can be tempting to make drastic and massive changes to our lives, as if that will help change take root more quickly. But unfortunately, that's not how sustainable change (let alone healing!) works. As much as we encourage you to *do* in this book, you will also be encouraged to rest. Because your body and your mind will need it, and only you know best when your body is able to take on something new. You may not be able to move on to the next chapter for a month, or more. There may be some exercises you look at and think, "I'll have to do that later" (or never!). All that we offer here are invitations and opportunities. You remain in control of your choices.

Breathe through it all. Consider the freedom inside these yet-unknown possibilities.

As much as we encourage you to do things alone, there will also be prompts that encourage you to connect what you're learning to being in community by sharing it with someone else. Again, this is not a process to be rushed, as relationship-building of any kind takes time, but we want you to know this now and be prepared for it, because connecting with people isn't something everyone may have practice in doing. But community is important. It is part of our Indigenous awareness, and an important part of what distinguishes the BCH process from the capitalist myth of "self-care" that the dominant society would have us believe. We (Adenike and Natasha) believe that we (humanity) are not meant to do any kind of work in isolation. Because if all of us are so intimately connected, at the cellular level, as we've previously stated, then it stands to reason that when one of us is wounded, all of us are. And, when one of us heals, healing may spread, just as knowledge does.

None of us individually knows everything. But every one of us knows *something*, and so we come together to share what we know and provide prompts to stir the knowing within you. Perhaps, as you process this knowing within yourself and with others around you, that sharing may resonate with them, and what they share may enhance your own healing and the healing of others around you, and that healing may spread. For helping professionals, particularly those who work with Black/African Diasporic peoples, this may transform your work in critically necessary ways. You may find yourselves personally changed and entering your sessions with more vulnerability and more comfort with the unknown. You may find yourselves opening the door to therapeutic relationships with more curiosity and humility and less attachment to the idea of you being any sort of "expert."

However you move through the world, we hope that this text helps you deepen your relationships, not just for the sake of those relationships but, in the context of community, for the sake of us all. Our collective liberation depends on it.

All material marked ★ are available to download for your own use at www.jkp.com/catalogue/book/9781805017684

Section 1

ANCESTRAL PERSPECTIVES ON HEALING AND CREATIVITY

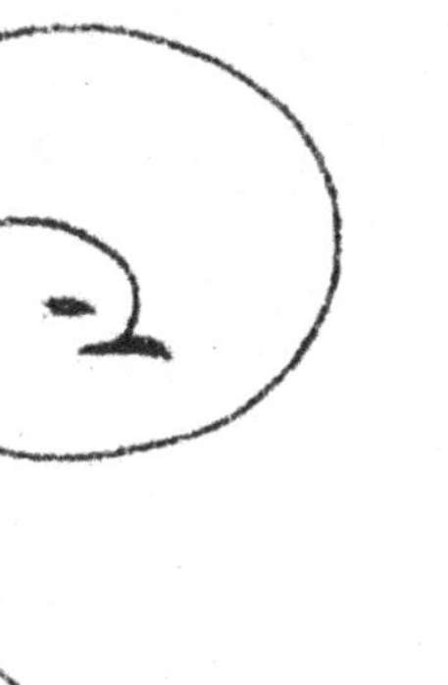

Chapter 1

To Heal, and to Create, is Liberatory

There is something about the word "healing" that equally excites and repulses people. As with most words and practices in any society, it holds all the history of how it has been used (or misused) and wielded (or weaponized) among us, most notably so on the most vulnerable among us. All this has an impact on the meaning we attach to the word, and idea of, healing.

We live in a western (Eurocentric, Christian-dominant, heteronormative, sexist, and ableist) world that tells us that if you are "defective" in any way, you are disposable. And what do people do when they are worried about being disposed of?

They hide.

We all do it. We are socialized to downplay any needs we may consider "weaknesses," or reframe them as strengths if we share them at all. Depending on how you were raised, you may have been led to believe that indicating any kind of need at all was dangerous, and thus to be avoided at all costs. For people with that kind of lived experience, which is common to many Black folks who descend from the lineages of chattel slavery and colonization, healing might be somewhat of a dirty word and something to be rejected, lest we be discarded: "I don't need healing! What, are you telling me I'm broken?!"

But what if we all are? What if everybody breaks sometimes? What if it wasn't such a stigmatized thing—to acknowledge that we all need healing now and then? That healing doesn't have to be a big thing with some kind of far-off destination but rather a natural and reflexive process, one that we can (and should expect to) undertake, again and again, as often as we may need it?

Of course, the beliefs and fears that lead us to resist stigmatization (of any kind!) come from a very real and complex place. That place lives in our bodies and memories, and we'll be spending a lot of time excavating that place throughout this book. But if we can start in this place, now, a place of realizing that healing is a thing we all need now and then, an opportunity arises: we have the chance to really look at ourselves and to define who (and how!) we truly are.

What are the various parts of ourselves that make us "us"? How do those parts motivate and/or repulse us and others? How have those parts been valued or weaponized, particularly against the most vulnerable among us? How can we re-member all of our whole and fullest selves?

As an example, I (Natasha) remember very vividly the moment I was first made aware of my Blackness in a tangible way, at a playdate surrounded by white children in North Dakota. Ironically it happened around the same time I became aware of myself as a Creative. In fact, both realizations actually came to me very similarly: someone else had to point them out to me.

There's a whole history of that as a phenomenon, isn't there? Someone you might know points out, "Hey, you know that's unique to you, right?" about some trait or practice of yours, long before you ever see that thing in yourself. Sometimes they're spot on, and sometimes they couldn't be further from the truth, particularly if you have been historically marginalized: other people often tell us who they think we are before we have the opportunity to name ourselves in our own bodies and words. Either way, the experience can be jarring.

In my case, the girl who pointed my Blackness out to me at a playdate in North Dakota didn't have any kind of accurate vocabulary for what I was. She simply refused to play with me because I was "dirty." I remember being so surprised by such a ridiculous idea until it dawned on me that, oh yeah, nobody else in this backyard looked like me but the people I was related to. This kid had probably never seen a Black person in real life before. Then I realized I'd never called myself that before: Black. Of course, I knew myself as a member of an Afro-Caribbean family. I knew that sense of belonging that came from being with my family, and others from our culture. But this was the first moment I felt othered by it, realizing that this thing—my Blackness—had more than one dimension to it, and that not every dimension was safe.

The initial feeling of realization is hard to describe. For me, I feel it in my chest, a sort of "opening up" that causes me to inhale—or is it the inhale that causes the sense of opening up? Then the muscles around my face relax, almost in relief at finally making sense of something my body/mind didn't even know it was trying to reconcile.

I felt all that in this moment, with my non-Black peer discovering my Blackness in the Great White North. I felt it when I first heard myself described as "creative" too. In that moment, however, I remember basking in that feeling. "You're so creative!" this person had said, and my chest filled up, my face relaxed, my whole body felt like it was opening and unfolding in the best of ways, like suddenly the whole world felt accessible to me.

Like I could fly.

Finding out about my Blackness in this way didn't feel like that. In that moment, surrounded by whiteness, and the disdain of this other child, the relief of realization was quickly filled with a sense of dampening, like it was not safe for me to let my guard down long enough to truly feel into what I was experiencing.

I don't usually tell people that part of the story. Sometimes I just let what that girl said and did hang in the air as the uncomfortable thing that it was, without elaboration on how I felt about any of it. Sometimes I go on to talk about how I sat down and explained to this kid that no, I wasn't dirty, this was my skin. Sometimes the color of my audience dictates how much of the thing needs to be shared and how I share it. Every choice like this is intended by me to be adaptive and protective, based on how safe I feel in the environment in which the story is being told. But even having to make that choice at all feels like a cage. Like I'm not really free if I'm having to think that hard about my safety in a room.

This, too, is a known phenomenon. In his book, *Whistling Vivaldi,*[1] researcher Claude M. Steele explores the theory of stereotype threat, which is the experience a person has when they are concerned they are going to be stereotyped. He recounts studies where mixed groups of individuals, from various genders and/or races, all previously identified to be high achievers in their area, be it mathematics, science, or athletics, are brought together to take some sort of test of their skill and all told, "Sometimes (insert minority peoples here) struggle with these concepts." In every one of those studies, when that phrase was heard by someone who came from a minoritized group, be it women, members of the LGBTQIA+ community, or Black/Indigenous People of Color (BIPOC), those individuals underperformed, and people from the more encouraged (dominant) group overperformed. Remember, all participants in these studies came in on equal footing, chosen for the study based on similar test scores and capabilities. But just being told, "You might be bad at this because of who you are," became a self-fulfilling prophecy for those who had been marginalized all their lives.

Stereotypes and stigma are wounds that have been built over generations of targeted and systemic abuse. And what we know of any wound is that if left unattended, it can fester, and infection can spread. Where there is infection, there is potential for loss of life or limb. The initial wound doesn't even need to be that big! Being nipped on your finger by a cat can kill you if the wound isn't cleaned and carefully bandaged or is otherwise not allowed to heal. And that is what we've seen in many Black communities—we continue to be wounded, and re-wounded, over and over again, by the initial horrors of colonization that have continued to evolve over time, from chattel slavery to Jim Crow and apartheid, from redlining and other racist forms of redistricting to gentrification, and other exploitative practices that still live today. White supremacy, to date, has never disappeared; it has just mutated into new forms, each more insidious than the last, festering in every place it has touched, even if all looks "resolved" on the surface.

The image at the top of this section is an interpretation by Natasha of what's known as the Sankofa bird.[2] This mythical creature and symbol comes from the people of Ghana and is commonly depicted as a bird looking over its back while carrying an egg, or a seed, in its mouth. The phrase frequently associated with this image is the translation of Sankofa, which means "go back and retrieve it." We use this image with intentionality and great awareness of its meaning. Our history is something we carry in our minds, and in our bodies. It informs the way we hold ourselves now, and how we move forward. You will see the image of this bird evolve as we progress through this book.

Let us remember in this moment that our Ancestors' legacies stretch beyond the histories of our traumas. Africa was the birthplace of countless civilizations. Our Ancestors created whole artforms and universities and were working with the gifts of their lands long before European colonizers came and decided to exploit them. We carry deep knowledge. Some of the oldest knowledge. We carry this wisdom alongside our trauma.

Still, trauma can be loud. And just like wisdom, it can come from many places.

If we can acknowledge that intergenerational trauma is present for groups of people harmed by large-scale events, we have to acknowledge that intergenerational trauma is also present for individuals and families who have experienced patterns of systemic and interpersonal abuse and neglect in various forms through their lineage.

The legacy of colonization is vast, and deep. Thus, our efforts to combat it must be even more expansive.

This is where creativity comes in. Creativity can include any and all thoughts/practices that invite questions or play. We are creative when we find ways to make small spaces hold many people and needs, creative when we crowdsource funds, creative when we make a few seemingly undesirable ingredients into a nourishing and satisfying meal. These are the forms of creativity that Black folks have had centuries of practice leveraging, to the point that they are almost innate to us now. Consider the mothers who packed meals for the people traveling to the Million Man March in Washington[3] [4] so they wouldn't have to stop as often in places that might not be safe as they traveled across the Jim Crow South. Consider the free breakfasts that the Black Panthers[5] fought to provide for their communities' children so that no child would have to go to school hungry. All the ways we have derived over time to "make a way out of no way." This is creativity.

Even so, we frequently hear people come into BCH spaces saying, "I don't know if I'd call myself a Creative, but I enjoy (insert XYZ artform) and I want to make space for more of that in my life." To statements like that, our response is always the same:

"That sounds like a Creative to me!"

There is a reason why people often feel so drawn to creative acts to infuse into their lives. Whether it's for a hobby, your day job, or something in between, to create something (anything!)—a thought becoming a sound, a gesture, or a word—is a freeing feeling. It is the act of bringing something into being and setting it on a path where it might take on a life of its own. This is also a very vulnerable act, because what is created comes from inside of us, and as such it is connected to our deepest feelings and sense of being in the world. To create something is to reveal something, and what is revealed may not always be experienced comfortably by all involved.

And yet creativity is intuitive. Our Ancestors were creative. Creativity is arguably part of our evolutionary process! We created tools, and those tools catalyzed new ways of being which have been intimately connected to our capacity for survival. Tools changed how we hunted, made it possible for us to begin farming, and changed how we ate. Tools also changed how we communicated and interacted with each other. We made instruments that expanded the foundation of what we now call music. And we made weapons, which led to terrifying and paradoxical innovations in war and medicine.

Sitting with these realities may bring up a lot of complicated feelings. They may challenge or enforce foundational beliefs that we each have about the world. When you do this work (the work of healing, catalyzed by creativity, and connecting to others through that process), you start to see things that may not previously have been clear; you start to see things as they are, or maybe on a deeper level than you ever imagined them to be. These things might be scary and undesirable. Looking at them makes us feel exposed and vulnerable in ways that we are not familiar with and that are deeply uncomfortable.

This is the paradox of healing: necessary and nourishing as it can be, it can also hurt to heal, and it isn't always easy. Healing also takes time. Our bodies and minds need that time—to digest, and to process, to become (re)acquainted with ourselves, over and over again. This is why we encourage you to take your time with this process.

This is also how healing becomes liberatory. As Audre Lorde said, "If I didn't define myself for myself, I would be crunched up into other people's fantasies of me and eaten alive."[6] Making the choice to face ourselves and make meaning from the many knowledges we are connected to, over and over, we grow into the fullest and most authentic forms of our own being, with balanced boundaries and mindfulness of how we are all interconnected; each of us drawing light from the affirming sun and water from deep wells of resilience, weaving upwards in collaboration, and sprouting through hardened soil. We become our truest selves, free to keep exploring and defining, and re-defining, what that is into infinity, without restriction.

Tap in for Reflection: Describe Sensations, Let Memory Support You

For our first reflection, we want to offer you a few ways to engage: you can scan the QR code to listen to Natasha reading the following prompts, or locate this exercise in the accompanying workbook, where prompts are provided with journaling space. Not every exercise will be coming with a QR like this going forward, but the workbook will continue to be a place for those who prefer things broken down into more bite-sized pieces.

Take a moment to name a **sensation** you feel in your body right now. This is different than an emotion. This is something to do with the way your **body** feels. It may be something that **informs** your emotions, but this is the thing that comes **before** your brain begins to interpret.

You can explore the sensation coming to your brain with your mind alone, or with a pen and paper. Words like "tired" may come to your mind first, or "tension"; any of that is ok! Whatever word you arrive at, write it down.

Now we're going to go deeper. Within any given word there are additional qualities worth excavating, because your definition of "tired" or "tense" may not be the same as someone else's. What is "tired" to you? Is it a heaviness in your eyelids or something you feel in other parts of your body? If you named "tension," where is it? Does it have a specific point of origin, or does it feel widespread? Is it a high level of tension or something you can release just by bringing awareness to it? This is the level of **specificity** we want to encourage here.

Once you've written your word, and added some specificity to its description, take a breath or two before going any further.

Can you remember another time you felt this way? Let yourself lightly explore the memory of the feeling, just for a moment. Let it be like a hologram around you, lightly projecting out of the corner of your eye, easy to disperse at will, otherwise immersive. A memory you can pause, rewind, or blow away.

Now shift your focus to an experience following that feeling—one where something (or someone) improved what you were experiencing, at any time, in a meaningful way. Let your senses lean in to that memory of **meaning**. What was happening to your skin, in response to the temperature, or other people or objects about you, wherever you were in that moment? What did the air smell like?

Take a moment to let this memory give you a **message**. As with most gifts, you don't really get to choose what you will receive. This message will be chosen for you as whatever thought first enters your head after you finish this sentence…

Whether this message came from your subconscious, the Holy Spirit, an Ancestor, or the most recent food to enter your digestive system, you will know this message to be unique to this moment. Sit with this moment; as you do this, knowing that if this feels hard or uncomfortable in any way, it is ok to stop, try again later, or move on. **You know your body/mind best** and can trust it to signal to you when it's time to change gears, in any direction.

Ok?

If/when you feel ready, let the message you received just now simmer within you for a bit. Play it back in your memory or read it aloud as many times as feels necessary for you to commit it to memory, such that it can autoplay in your mind while you feel deeper into your body. Set a timer if you feel the need to contain the experience in some way. Again, you know your body/mind best. **Pay attention** to what happens within you as the message simmers.

What does your breath feel like right now? What else might be happening in your body right now? And how might it relate to the sensation you made note of earlier?

Take a moment to jot down anything that has shifted in your body in response to this experience. Then, **step away** from this book for a time. Go for a walk, get a drink of water or some food to eat, and let what you've experienced marinate. The work will still be here when you get back, and you'll be better equipped on the other side of a break.

Part of the dominant educative process many of us undergo in western countries involves a sort of prioritization (maybe even a deification?) of "objectivity," or "fact": that which can be "proven" or defined with quantifiable measurements. A byproduct (or perhaps it is a feature?) of this type of emphasis on the quantifiable is that it devalues the felt senses, the parts of us that make meaning from what we perceive around us. That is what the exercise you just completed is built to complicate. You could complete it 1200 times and have 1200 unique experiences, each with a unique meaning to you, a single human sharing the planet with billions of other humans. Even if many humans might share the same thought, there is no way of knowing for certain how the things you **sense or feel** on any given day might be interacting with someone else's life, or the meaning that may or may not be made there by that exact moment.[7]

The Gradient of Potential Is Infinite. Facts Aren't Everything

There is always more that our bodies can tell us, or guide us to do, if we are able to listen and make sense of their cues.

Yet we are often taught that our own bodies and minds cannot be trusted, making it easier to ignore the larger reality of how every body/mind throughout time has had feelings and senses that guided their actions, whether they were aware of them or not. Ignoring our body/mind in this way dulls us to our own capacity for more complex ways of being in and responding to our world. It makes us easier to manipulate.

Better you be the one holding the reins of your own body/mind (as much as any one person can hold the reins of anything so expansive) than anyone else.

What you were invited to do just now was to lay out the ingredients of a "power up" for your brain: you have the memory of the first feeling you were invited to describe and the memory of it improving, and then you have meaning (a message) made from weaving them together in your body/mind. Now, the next time you feel whatever you were feeling when you first began this exercise, your body will have one more thread of connection between that feeling and the one that improved it. Were you to practice this act of tapping in and remembering more often—on your own, by yourself, for yourself—those connections would grow even stronger.

Your own gradient of potential will shine brighter.

Even if all that comes to your mind at this moment is a vague sense of familiarity with the metaphor of "power ups," this is the gift of imagination! Creatively assorted words made you feel/remember things!

Now imagine this as a healing practice. In the remembering of a time when something got better, you are (re)creating the conditions for it to get a little better now, too.

Creativity, of any kind, makes space for us to go deeper into ourselves: our motivations, our intentions, our impacts, and other realities of who and where we are in the world, and in our lives. This kind of space-making yields more qualitative, deeply rooted, and sustaining results. These are toolsets that humanity so needs to strengthen at this moment.

Our current society isn't so big on giving people space. Our every free moment of time, energy, and attention are constantly lapped at by stimuli in order to produce, or spend, capital. Let the machine be without you for a moment. You may find you want more for yourself.

Kindle Your Inner Traveler

Part of what will get us to that more strengthened place humanity needs is to be as precise as we can be with ourselves, not just about who/where/how we are but also about what motivates us toward making things better for ourselves or others. Even better if we can do this from an honest (real) and grounded place that can clearly see and draw meaning from the relationship between who/where/how we are now and any other place we might hope to reach. Being real about where we are can help building a map to our wholeness that much easier. But it may also bring us into awareness of just how far we are from the places we hope to be, and that can sometimes be hard. Be gentle with yourself as you explore these places. Important things happen in the time it takes to really sit with how it feels to be where you are, beyond the intellectual sense of, "Oh, I feel sad about that, bummer." When you get to know your feelings, deeply, at the level of specificity with which we asked you to define whatever sensation you lifted in the above reflective process, you are training yourself to recognize the warning signs of those feelings more efficiently, long before the point of festering. Remember what we know of wounds: sometimes time is all that stands between someone losing a limb, or their life. Healers sometimes have to make split-second decisions. But those decisions come from time—sometimes decades!—spent building awareness and knowledge; the kind of time and awareness we are asking you to dedicate and build in this book. Becoming aware of sadness, tiredness, stress, tension, whatever it is, as something that lives not just in your mind but also in your body, might just save you and your loved ones a world of hurt someday, even if it feels scary or painful now.

This is the cost of liberation, and of healing: to face fear and pain, to come to know them and everything they touch, intimately. This includes how they show up in your life, what they feel like, sound like, look like, so much so that you can begin to more readily recognize their impacts and move through them to become more whole and more free.

And, again, we have to be real: there is no way to know what wholeness will look like in the end, for any of us. Some people heal with minimal scarring, while some are not so lucky.

Can you accept this uncertainty?

Some people are able to heal in ways that easily cascade into the lives of others around them. Their people see and accept the way their loved one is changing with open arms. Others find themselves losing people on their healing journey—people for whom the changes emerging in the person they thought they knew are simply too much to handle. It is important to be aware of these possible outcomes.

Breathe.

As we process these possibilities, we recognize that within every risk we name, there may also be a reward; for instance, scar tissue, while painful, can help us to remember to move with care, lest we reinjure ourselves. And losing people, while painful, can sometimes make space for more fulfilling relationships to thrive. Even the most subtle increase in awareness can promote critically necessary changes—in our perception of self, in our dreams, hopes, bodies, personalities, skills, and relationships. In each shift there is a new dimension of space for us to create and grow into. In that space there may be lessons that we need to learn so that we can utilize the newfound space in ourselves most responsibly/effectively. There may also be realities that space allows us to see more clearly, people or practices that we may need to let go of to make room for even more of ourselves to expand. Here, in the potential for even more creativity and space-making, is where liberation begins to bloom.

For me (Natasha) some of what I have had to let go of has been a great deal of shame, much of which has been attached to being perceived as "naive" or "gullible." I have always been deeply sensitive, a fiercely hopeful and trusting person, even in the face of people who have abused me or otherwise did not deserve my trust. I have had to sit with those pieces of myself, to hold my experiences (and myself!) gently, look them/me in the eye, and release the shame to find where my deepest and truest self lies: the part of me that knows I have *never* deserved to be harmed and, in fact, that *no one ever deserves to be harmed.* In that process, I have found discernment and agency in myself, a way to hone my sensitivities, and to target my hope and trust in directions that are more rooted in my own values, and the gifts I have been given that have contributed to the me that feels most alive—the most whole. So for me, if I were to put this into table form, my risks and rewards might look like this:

Risks of healing for Natasha	Potential rewards for Natasha
Shame Judgment Fear of being wounded (again) Heightened sensitivity	Greater discernment Stronger sense of agency Stronger sense of hope Manageable sensitivities More rooted and clear values alignment More attunement with creative and intuitive gifts More wholeness

I (Adenike) had to learn that the parts of myself that I had ignored and avoided had value. I had to (and am still trying to!) let go of the myth of perfection—good enough really is good enough! Coming into my healing is a process of self-discovery and self-acceptance on a deeper level than I could have ever thought. I am learning that my specific ways of being creative, of understanding things, of sharing information, of building relationships are all valid. I can let go of having a persona that I think my profession or my society expects me to be. This is where some semblance of balance, and nuance, also comes into play. For while I strive now to avoid being dependent on others in ways that would strip me of my own agency, I am deeply aware of the value of community and of how much humans need each other to survive. Healing is not something that can ever, truly, be done alone. Our Ancestors knew this.

Risks of healing for Adenike	Potential rewards for Adenike
Having to face parts of myself I may not like Not being "perfect" anymore Feeling "dependent" on others	Self-acceptance Re-defined sense of validity More authentic being Deeper relationship with community

What might your own table of risks and rewards look like?

Note: If you are a helping professional, or part of a family or community with others you think may benefit from these experiences, you may feel tempted to bring this exercise to someone you work or live with without having first undertaken it yourself. We urge you to complete these exercises for *you*, before bringing them to anyone else. Part of what this work is meant to do is to bring you into a deeper relationship with your own self, in order to open up the space/possibility for deeper connections that will, of course, eventually expand beyond you, but we don't want to rush that process! So, we encourage you to really sit with these invitations for self-exploration and not rush into using these exercises with anyone else until you have done them yourself.

Pour into Practice: Calculate Your "Risks and Rewards"

What are the risks of healing for you? What are the potential rewards? List them below.

Risks of healing (things you may need to work through or let go of):	**Potential rewards:**

Remember, take your time with this. Some responses may arrive quickly and with great clarity. Others may emerge more slowly (if at all), and with more nuance and gray areas. It's all possible!

Now let's bring in some creativity!

Remember, perfection is not the point. Our Ancestors were creative, and so are you. Creativity can begin with the simplest of actions. For this moment, let's focus on a short series of choices. You will want to have some colored pens/pencils, crayons, or markers near you for this.

1. Identify one word from each of the columns you have created: one risk and one reward.
2. Center your focus on the risk you have chosen. You are going to ask yourself a question about that word. The question is not about what the word means in any literal sense. The question is going to be about choosing a symbol to represent that word.
3. The symbol you choose is going to be a color or a texture. When you look at the risk you have chosen, what color or texture rises in your mind? Let the color/texture become vibrantly clear in your mind. It might help you to say your word, color, or texture aloud as you sit with it.
4. Place that color or texture next to the word it represents in your list. You may wish to outline or highlight your word in the color you chose, or make some other representation, like a wavy or jagged line to indicate texture. Remember, your symbol does not have to be perfect! You are simply making a choice to make meaning in some small way. This is a creative act!
5. When you have completed the representation of your symbol next to your risk word, repeat this series of actions/choices for the word you've chosen on your rewards list.
6. Afterwards, sit for a minute or two with any feelings that may have arisen for you as you chose these symbols. You may wish to journal these feelings, sit with them further, or breathe them out and go on with your day. Any/all of

these feelings and decisions are ok! Recognize them and let them flow as they will, without judgment.

Note: There are many ways this experience can be adapted. You may wish to try out other kinds of symbols, like sound or gesture. Whatever you choose, resist the urge to create something complicated or lengthy. Let it be simple; let it be small, like spelling out the letters of your risk or reward in its color/texture, focusing closely on every stroke, every little detail that you make. Let yourself find satisfaction in the infinite potential of one choice at a time.

This may be a vulnerable experience for you. You may feel self-conscious or silly. The world we live in today is one that moves fast and with lots of complexity. And yet we are all connected to Ancestors who once lived in a time before we counted seconds on a clock. Letting yourself sit with simplicity is not just for simplicity's sake or being satisfied with "less"; it is about making space for great things to emerge from (seemingly) small spaces.

Remember, even if you are physically alone as you do this, you are never *truly* alone. You are connected, right now, to someone else, somewhere else. By blood or proximity, by time, or by space. You are connected to resources, right now, even if you can't perceive them. Let these truths give you strength to sit with any difficult thoughts or feelings that may arise.

You are building towards something important. You are building towards the version of yourself that is most whole and most able to leverage the connections and capacity already within you, regardless of whether your conscious mind is yet aware of their existence or potential.

Chapter 2

The Wounds We Need to Heal—Intergenerational and Race-based Trauma

We are all, at this point, well aware that there is more to our bodies than meets the eye. From a biological standpoint, we know that there are millions of organelles within millions of cells that make up our organs and systems. We know that there is an incredible amount of information coded on the chromosomes that determine the color of our eyes, the amount of curl in our hair, and whether our voice sounds just like our great-grandfather's. We understand that our bodies can carry traits that, when given the optimal environment for expression, can lead us to develop conditions like cancer. Our bodies carry the effects of gene mutations from many generations back. And we know that these physiological traits aren't the only things our bodies carry.

Intergenerational trauma affects many different racial and ethnic groups around the world. Key examples are the descendants of people who survived the Holocaust, descendants of Alaska Native and American Indian communities that faced war and genocide from European colonizers, and descendants of Black people in the United States who have experienced systemic oppression and mass incarceration.[1 2 3] When we look at the last group of people mentioned—Black people in the United States—we can see that events that occurred over 400 years ago have long-reaching effects that have significant impact on how folks live and engage in contemporary society. To get a sense of what that looks like, we'll present a timeline of major events and experiences for Black people in the United States, beginning with their arrival as enslaved Africans and ending with the present day. This timeline is a basic overview; it would be beyond the scope of this book to list everything in detail.

Even though this timeline and other examples or experiences we share are based in the United States where we live, it is crucial to remember that intergenerational and race-based trauma as a result of colonialism and slavery are very much present in other places like Central and South America, the Caribbean, parts of Western Africa, and among the descendants of African and Caribbean people living in the United Kingdom and beyond. While the account that follows focuses on Black life in the United States, many aspects of that experience are similar to what members of the African Diaspora across the world have in their lineages and bodies.

A note before we embark on this timeline: we are going to do our utmost to cradle descriptions of intergenerational and race-based traumas with care. This means we will, wherever possible, keep descriptions of violence or other traumatic events brief and limited to an intensity level of 5 or lower (on a scale of 1 to 10), with little to no explicit detail. Even with this care, we recognize that any discussion of trauma can be activating for our bodies/minds, so we will be easing in and out of this particular historical discussion of trauma by using a fictional family as a focal point for identifying—on a surface level—how trauma can show up and be tended to in Black households. We'll call this family the Weavers. Some of these familial elements may feel familiar to readers, and some may not. Some of what you will read may activate memories/sensations for you, and some may not. Remember, any sense of intensity will eventually pass, and you know your body/mind best. We'll remind you to tap in and check with any part of you that may need tending to as we go. Be sure to take those breaks where you need to!

INTRODUCING THE WEAVERS

Cara and Ben are two Black, married, recently retired elders. Each one has multiple siblings still living, though both sets of their parents are gone. Their own four children are grown, some with children of their own. Some live geographically close to each other. Some live further away. Each child has a deep and complex relationship with their parents, and with each other.

Despite the complexity of their relationships, the Weavers take great care in finding time to be together at least once a year. Those who live further away will travel to visit those who live closer together. This creates somewhat of an imbalance, as those folks who live closer together frequently find themselves playing host to those who travel from further away, and those who live further away find themselves spending money on travel to reach those who live closer together. As a result of this, there are occasional tensions in the family that can surface as bickering or bitterness between siblings. Cara typically becomes very distressed whenever she hears of her children bickering and will often call each of them anxiously in succession upon hearing of any discontent, to remind each of her kids that, "All we got is each other," and, "Family is family." These calls are tolerated by her children but rarely appreciated. Everyone tends to leave those calls feeling frustrated.

The Weavers are descended from enslaved African peoples who were abducted from their home countries in the period of time known as the Maafa, or "The Great Tragedy" of chattel slavery.

Chattel Slavery: 1600s–1865

Slavery has been part of many cultures, like Ancient Greece and Ancient Rome, and even within some African cultures. The difference between those forms of slavery and the type practiced in the United States and other parts of the Americas is that people who were enslaved outside of Euro-colonial structures had legal status and were able to buy their freedom, marry, and even gain citizenship. It's interesting to note that it was only when Europeans began the push to gain wealth and power through global colonization that Black Africans were seen as "lacking" essential human qualities, thus making them "naturally fitted" to the role of being enslaved.[4] The chattel slavery prevalent in the Americas allowed white European-descended people to exploit, injure, torment, and torture African-descended people with impunity. The degradation and subjugation experienced by enslaved Africans upon arrival in the United States led to the disruption of family structures; increased infant mortality; physical, sexual, and emotional abuse; limited access to medical care and food resources; and few opportunities to act with agency.[5] Most likely, many enslaved people experienced symptoms of post-traumatic stress disorder such as depression, anxiety, suicidality, and grief.[6] As these Africans had children, it is also likely that these children would have experienced a lack of parental support and care (as their enslaved parents were either incapacitated or kept from caring for their children). Many families were broken apart when children and parents were sold and separated from each other, never to see each other again. One of the first things newly emancipated African-Americans did after the end of the Civil War was to search for family members from whom they had been separated. There were many notices in newspapers sharing details about loved ones and asking for any possible information.

> Any family can have complicated relationships or imbalances in how their primary way of spending time together is being experienced by various members of the group. Knowing that the Weavers are descended from the Maafa, however, lends a particular meaning to phrases like, "All we got is each other."
>
> Imagine that one day, when Cara calls one of her and Ben's adult children to remind them that, "Family is family," that her child has recently spent some time exploring their family's history and has an awareness of how the trauma of chattel slavery has encoded into their bodies. They know that a deep layer of their mother's anxiety response may include messages encoded from that time, even if they're just perceptions, of threats like lifelong separation. So, that day, this child—let's call them Shae—disrupts the usual frustrating path of these conversations with their mother by asking, "Mom, can we take a deep breath together? I think we're both feeling anxious and I want us both to be in a more grounded place." Shae has made a choice to tend with care to a possible trauma response, introducing the potential for healing a generational wound with deep origins.

Reconstruction, Sharecropping, and the Great Migration: 1865–1954

The years following slavery in the United States were filled with equally harrowing times. Although Black people were granted citizenship status during the Reconstruction era (1865–1877) and could enter into public life, they were not always treated as equals or granted access to economic opportunity to the same degree white citizens were. Yes, there were instances of Black people becoming members of state and federal legislatures, owning businesses, opening colleges, and becoming professionals, but they were still subjected to discrimination and grave harm. In many Southern states, formerly enslaved people were able to rent land from their former enslavers. Payment took the form of surrendering a percentage of their harvest to their landlords. This practice was known as sharecropping, and continued into the 1940s. Often, these arrangements were not equitable and resulted in cycles of debt and impoverishment.

For those Black people in Southern towns who were perceived as too successful, or as making too much of a stir regarding civil rights, there was the threat of lynching. Lynching was a means to terrorize and control Black communities. The Equal Justice Initiative's report on lynching in the United States identifies more than 4000 instances of Black men, women, and children being brutally tortured, their bodies put on display for white and Black people to see, to remind everyone of their places in society.[7] From the 1880s to 1940s, the widespread practice of lynching made it increasingly difficult for Black people to live as full citizens in the United States. As government and state officials did not effectively hold accountable those who committed lynchings, many Black communities lived in fear and were inhibited from living out the promises of emancipation. Ultimately, many Black people left Southern towns to move to urban areas in the North and West, a period known as the Great Migration (1910–1970). While such a move may have allowed survival, people still faced discrimination in the form of being relegated to living in lower-resourced areas and prohibited from living in more affluent suburban areas (redlining), being excluded from higher-paying jobs, and being seen as criminal elements by white people unused to living with Black people.[8] [9]

Cara and Ben currently live in Detroit, Michigan, in a predominantly Black neighborhood of people whose families traveled there during the Great Migration. Ben's family migrated after the burning of Black Wall Street in 1921. Black Wall Street was a name given to the Greenwood district of Tulsa, Oklahoma, a previously thriving community of Black businesses, houses, churches, and schools.[10] When one of the Black Greenwood residents was suspected of sexually assaulting a white woman, 35 city blocks of this community were destroyed by a white mob. The mob killed 300 people, injuring 800, and leaving 9000 without homes. Law enforcement did little to curb the violence and, in fact, arrested and detained Black men and not any of the white mob. Ben's maternal grandfather was among those who experienced this trauma as a young man, though Ben does not recall him ever speaking of the incident. All he knows about it came from his maternal grandmother, who would use it to explain why his grandfather would become so agitated by loud or startling noises, often yelling at whoever was responsible for them. Grandma would say, "When your grandpa gets startled, it's like his body is remembering those bad times."

To this day, Ben has a habit of calling out, "Sorry!" whenever he makes a loud noise, wherever he is. This is a coping mechanism he inherited from his mother, who developed it to try and mitigate her father's trauma response to startling sounds. Various non-Black friends of the family have noticed that Ben does this and are curious about why. One day Trina, another of the Weaver's adult children, has a conversation with her sibling Shae about the impact of race-based trauma on their family, and their father's inherited coping mechanism comes up. They wonder together about whether making a trip to Tulsa sometime might provide an opportunity for them to learn more about what happened to their great-grandfather there and maybe make some connections with other descendants of that time.

Incidents of violence like the burning of Black Wall Street were ways to remind Black people of their perceived inferiority to white people and that their advancement in society would not be tolerated. Just a few days after the riot, the mayor of Tulsa established a committee to oversee rebuilding in Greenwood, zoning the district for increased industrial development. Many survivors were offered a pittance for their land and relegated to less suitable places to live. Although in 1997 the Tulsa Reparations Coalition was established to investigate the events of the 1921 riot and to identify actions to take as restitution, not much has been done to offer financial compensation to survivors and their descendants.

Do you see it, straining against the facade of our "post-racial" world? This is deep and tender scar tissue.

Breathe.

Tap in for Reflection: Describe Sensations (Again!)
Check in with your body. Make note of any sensations that feel important to name, or to address. If you're feeling tension, take a moment to breathe or stretch. If you're feeling hungry or thirsty, or tired, meet those needs as best you can before moving ahead to the next passage.

Jim Crow: 1954–1968

During the period from the end of the Civil War to the height of the Civil Rights Movement in the 1960s, "Jim Crow" laws governed the lives of Black people in harsh ways. Jim Crow was the name of a character in a 19th-century minstrel song. He was a formerly enslaved Black person usually portrayed as unintelligent and shiftless, and represented by white men who painted their faces black. Mainly enforced in the South, Jim Crow laws were used to keep Black communities from registering to vote and from owning or holding on to inherited land, and to force them into a segregated existence. This effectively prohibited them from being treated as equals and having access to the same rights, privileges, and resources as their white counterparts.

After World War II, things started to shift, as with the United States taking center stage as the "leader of the free world," the moral superiority of American policy would be called out if Black citizens were actively oppressed and discriminated against at all levels of American society. In the 1950s, actions like the Montgomery Bus Boycott and the court ruling of Brown vs. The Board of Education started to dismantle some of the institutional infrastructure that kept racism legal. Actions like these were not readily welcomed in many Southern states, and many tried to preserve the status quo through creating local laws in direct contradiction to Supreme Court mandates and through the terrorism of groups like the Ku Klux Klan.

In the face of this, the Civil Rights Movement took shape, with Black and non-Black students, church leaders, members of the National Association for the Advancement of Colored People (NAACP), and political leaders gathering, educating, marching, registering Black voters, and protesting to make justice and equality a reality. In 1964, the Civil Rights Act was passed, making it illegal to deny access to public accommodations, employment, and federal-supported programs based on race, color, religion, sex, and national origin. A year later, the Voting Rights Act was passed, to end racial discrimination in voter registration and elections, followed by the Fair Housing Act, ending discrimination in housing, in 1968. Throughout the 1960s, civil rights leaders, including Dr. Martin Luther King, Jr., pursued justice at the intersection of race and class, calling for improved economic opportunity for poor Black folks and other non-Black people who experienced poverty. By the end of the decade, there were more legal provisions in place to safeguard the rights of Black people as citizens in the United States. Behind each provision exists a universe of stories and experiences: trauma and healing continuing to share paradoxical space.

> Three of the Weaver siblings—Trina, Shae, and another we'll call Mike—end up connecting in Tulsa, armed with some family history they received from extended family members on their father's side. Trina and Shae decide to make a road trip of it, retracing the highways that their family traversed when they made their Great Migration north. Along the way, the siblings stop at significant landmarks from their family's story, including a restaurant that a great-aunt recalls lining up outside for a rest stop and a drink from a segregated water fountain. The aunt recalls how seeing and speaking to other

Black folks from the road was part of how her family knew it was safe to stop at that particular site, even though the risk of violence was ever present. Shae takes photos at each remembered stop.

Mike recently moved to a suburb close to Tulsa, after living on the East Coast, and—as one of the siblings who usually has to travel for family gatherings—is excited to host his siblings at his home, where he lives with his partner and their kids. The fourth Weaver sibling was unable to make the trip due to obligations with their own growing family.

The Weaver siblings take one day to get settled at Mike's house, talking extensively over dinner as they share photos and compare notes from their family members' stories. They map out a plan for the next few days—of places they want to visit and people or organizations they want to get connected with while they're in town. Mike shares how he took the job that brought him to the Tulsa area after a long period of deliberation with his non-Black partner, because both knew the Weaver family's history with the region was traumatic and that living there might bring up a lot of complicated feelings. In the end, Mike states that he felt it was an important move for them, because he had recently started therapy and wanted to get more in touch with his roots in a different way than he had tried before. Shae makes particular note of this revelation from their brother and suggests that they try to find time to video call later with the sibling that wasn't able to make the trip, because maybe she might find it meaningful to be part of more conversations like this.

Post Civil Rights Movement—Present Day

The decade after the passing of the Civil Rights Act saw mixed results as legislators and activists across the United States attempted to make equality a reality. The continued push for desegregating schools and the increased development of affirmative action policies began to unnerve and anger poor white people in cities and towns that saw a blurring of lines and mingling of cultures. Black people were seen as significantly less intelligent, lazier, more inclined to live off welfare, and more prone to violence than white folks or other racial/ethnic minorities.

Political leaders found ways to reframe events to suggest that the Civil Rights Movement was about destroying law and order and promoting criminal behavior. Michelle Alexander notes how the progression of this narrative resulted in the creation of policies by presidents like Richard Nixon and Ronald Reagan calling for a war on drugs.[11] These policies promoted actions like increased policing of poor urban communities (home to primarily Black/Indigenous People of Color [BIPOC]) and harsher criminal sentences for possession of recreational and illegal drugs. By equating Blackness with criminality in the minds of the voting white public, the laws and attitudes of the Jim Crow era morphed into a new use of the criminal justice system that led to the mass incarceration of Black men—a new Jim Crow.

The disruptive, devastating, and destructive impact of mass incarceration over the past four decades is felt across many Black communities in the United States. There are roughly 5 million people in jails and prisons in the United States, nearly 2 million of whom are Black. This is an increase of about 500% since the 1970s.[12] [13] Contrary to popular belief, the rates of incarceration do not line up with increased rates of crime but more with changes in laws, policies, and sentencing. Policies like "stop and frisk" and variable approaches to sentencing on drug-related charges have been noted to target Black people and Indigenous and other people of color more than white people.[14] [15] [16] Despite the passing of laws banning discrimination, Black citizens in the United States (and also in the United Kingdom from the 1960s onwards) have routinely experienced increased instances of incarceration, increased likelihood of conviction of crime, and increased instances of police brutality and lack of support from the criminal justice system.[17] [18]

While prisons saw an overrepresentation of Black people, they were underrepresented in many other spaces, despite policies like affirmative action. Throughout the last three decades, there have been record numbers of Black people being passed over for jobs and housing.[19] [20] Although Black college student enrollment in Predominantly White Institutions (PWIs) increased in the 1970s, recent data shows a decline, especially at schools that no longer use race as a factor in admissions.[21] With the United States Supreme Court ruling in 2023 that effectively stopped the use of affirmative action policies, there is a growing possibility that Black student enrollment in college will continue to decline. Whether attending a PWI or starting a new job, there is never any guarantee that a Black individual will feel welcomed or supported. The experience of racism can range from microaggressions (subtle, usually unintentional insults, invalidations, and slights towards members of minoritized groups) to violent interactions, each incident further activating the trauma already remembered by our bodies.

Here we remember that our bodies and minds, and our Ancestors' legacies, are expansive, and responsive to tending, with care.

On day two of their trip, the Weaver siblings visit the place where their great-grandfather used to live as a child. The house no longer stands at that particular intersection—in fact, the area is rather hard to reach, but the siblings know it from another landmark given to them by one of their extended family members' stories.

As the siblings stand on the sidewalk approaching the location, Trina is caught off guard by a sudden urge to cry. Unbeknownst to her other siblings, there is a tightness in her chest, her cheeks flush, and her eyes water. When the siblings stop at the street corner across from the location they know to have once been their great-grandfather's front yard, Trina bursts into tears. While both of her other siblings are caught off guard by this, their instinctive reaction is to embrace their sister, and the three of them stand on the corner for a moment, gripping each other tightly.

When Trina's tears begin to subside, she pushes back from her siblings, lightly squeezing each of their shoulders in thanks, and then shakes her hands out in front of her body rapidly, with a deep inhale and exhale, shifting her weight on her toes like a boxer for a moment. Her siblings recognize this as one of Trina's somatic (body-based) exercises from a community care workshop she had told them she was taking, and turn to face their family's former yard as she finishes. Trina takes a few deep breaths, one hand on her chest, the other on her abdomen, then comes to stand beside her siblings again. She takes out her phone and snaps a photo of the abandoned lot across the street.

Race-Based and Intergenerational Trauma Have Impacts: So Does Healing

Black life in the United States is complicated. Black culture is equally appreciated and appropriated. Black public figures are equally celebrated and condemned, especially if they use their status to call attention to injustice and oppression against Black people.[22] [23] The 2010s saw activism increase in the light of greater sharing on social media of police brutality towards Black people. The Black Lives Matter Movement, a response to the dehumanizing effect of that brutality, has been mocked, ridiculed, and condemned in many spaces and revered in others. Recent political discourse and federal policy that disparages efforts to promote diversity, equity, inclusion, and belonging has increased fears that Black federal employees, scholars, educators, healthcare workers, community organizers, and activists could lose their livelihoods and maybe even their lives.

In the face of constant discrimination and misunderstanding, while navigating the normal ups and downs of life, Black people have been carrying the psychological weight and wounds of generations. Trauma can be passed epigenetically (i.e., through exposure to maladaptive behaviors like substance abuse and other forms of relational abuse) and psychologically (i.e., through the stories told about trauma that can cause the hearers to feel traumatized). Behaviors and practices that enslaved Africans used to survive their enslavement have been passed on through lineages, becoming ways of being in the world. Resmaa Menakem notes, "When these strategies are repeated and passed on over generations, they can become the standard responses in families, communities, and cultures." He continues by saying when multiple families and communities do this, "[[w]hen these] same strategies get internalized and passed down over generations within a particular group, it can start to look like culture."[24]

In 2000, David Williams and Ruth Williams-Morris reviewed the literature in the United States that discussed the effects of racism on mental health in Black people.[25] What they found indicates that the effects of institutional racism (i.e., racism enshrined in laws, policies, systems, and practices) as well as interpersonal racism can result in decreased quality of life; a decreased sense of self-worth and agency, resulting in depression, stress, anxiety, high blood pressure, and cardiovascular disease; anticipatory stress when identifying coping strategies for dealing with possible negative interactions with police; and a diminished sense of emotional, physical, and economic stability and security due to the impact of criminal activity in low-resourced communities. Even though this review was published over 25 years ago, there is still a need for legal, social, communal, and individual strategies to effectively address the conditions mentioned in those studies.

As I (Adenike) pause to review the timeline, I am aware of how much I've tried to limit my emotional responses to what I wrote and read. When I first wrote this, I was in the middle of the busyness of my day, going from one meeting and task to another. It wasn't until the next day when I was reflecting on a heated and intense interaction with my spouse that I realized that my body had suppressed my reactions to the harm and pain I had been immersing myself in as I wrote. I unfairly, and unknowingly, used conversation with my spouse as an avenue for discharging and unleashing that stored up hurt. As many times as I have seen documentaries and movies or read books and articles about slavery and racism, I am learning that I am not immune to the trauma they highlight. Trying to keep these events as facts in the same way that I would acknowledge that the sky is blue minimizes their significance and prevents me from finding helpful ways of experiencing and processing my feelings. Sitting with ugly, painful truths is no fun, but it is necessary if I want to identify effective ways of healing. I need to remember to give myself grace and space, to give my siblings in the Diaspora grace and space, as we reckon with history in order to heal.

In 400 years, Black people in the United States have faced indescribable horrors. And yet we survive, and thrive. Our Ancestors did not only pass on their traumas; they passed on their wisdom, their creativity, their artistry, their ingenuity, their beauty, their faith, their righteous rage, their humor, their guidance, and their love. By intentionally returning to those gifts and grounding ourselves in the truth of Black worthiness, we can change what we pass on to future generations.

It is the day before Trina and Shae are to depart from the Tulsa area, and the day that the Weaver siblings have all managed to coordinate a video call with their one sibling (who we'll call Janelle) that couldn't make the trip.

Janelle sits in her living room on the other side of the country, with her seven-year-old appearing on and off camera periodically, both of them marveling at the photos and stories being shared. She knows her child is curious about the history they're discussing and does her best to respond to questions from her little one with age-appropriate details. Mike, whose children are younger than Janelle's, makes a mental note of some of her framing, appreciating the way she describes how "hard memories can sometimes live in our bodies, but talking about them with people you love can help."

At some point, Janelle's child disappears off camera again and returns sometime later with a picture they have drawn of their great-great-grandfather waving from (or perhaps at?) his house on one side, while his great-grandchildren smile and wave from the other side of the street. Seeing this, the Weaver siblings all ooh and ah over the little one's talent, while Janelle presses a slightly tearful kiss to the top of her child's head. This kiss doesn't go unnoticed by the other Weavers, who proceed to shout over each other about who's going to give and receive the biggest hugs and kisses the next time they all see each other! Janelle says that she will make sure they bring the picture their child made when they next visit, as part of a way to continue the conversation with their parents and extended family.

The Weaver family demonstrates trauma responses and coping strategies that may be very familiar to many Black families: generational anxiety around family separation, heightened startle responses, and other somatic reactions to embodied memories. These are all behaviors that any one of us might have witnessed or engaged in ourselves. Therapy and community care workshops are just some of the ways these needs can be tended to. We will explore many more in this book! The care and affection we envision between the Weavers, and their commitment to continued conversations and exploration of what is emerging for each of them, as they delve deeper into their family history, together, is something we wish for us all.

Tap in for Reflection: Revisit Your Memories, Risks, and Rewards

Check in with your body again, making note of any sensations and meeting any needs. Then revisit that memory of meaning from the reflection where we first invited you to describe sensations, "Tap in for Reflection: Describe Sensations, Let Memory Support You" and remember a time when someone or something improved the situation you were in, in some way.

Take a moment to recall the sensations of the meaning you made (any scents, sounds, etc.) as you revisit that memory and the memory of the message you received from it.

Consider: What value might the meaning that the Weavers are making on their trip (with the photos they're taking, stories they're telling, physical interactions they are having, etc.) be having on their bodies in these first few days? What value might you imagine that it holds for them down the road, years later? Generations later?

Now take a moment to revisit your own list of risks and rewards in relation to your personal healing journey, and update the rewards list with anything you've named above that you hadn't previously listed there.

Check in with your body once again, and take another break, if need be.

Hopefully, each time you do this, the transitions between checking in, naming sensations, making meaning, and documenting what emerges are beginning to feel smoother and more easeful to do. If not, that's ok! And if it feels like any changes you're experiencing are incremental, that's ok too! In fact, that's probably for the best—remember, small, incremental changes are more sustainable. Continue to be patient with yourself!

Chapter 3

Creative Healing Is Ancestral Work

There is a lineage of lived experiences from our Ancestors, which come into our lives in different ways—some seem helpful, some less so—and then we become Ancestors for future generations. Thus, it becomes an act of care and service to attend to our own sense of wholeness, for those who will come after us. In this way, to quote Layla F. Saad, we are working towards becoming "better Ancestors."[1]

The idea of healing has been present in my (Adenike's) life for almost as far back as I can remember. My grandmother was a nurse. Her brother was a doctor. My mother was a doctor. Several of her cousins are doctors and nurses. Attending to the wounds and illnesses of the body was part of their way of keeping loved ones and their communities whole. Looking back, I realize that even though they never explicitly spoke about healing emotional wounds, the way they approached their acts of tending to physical ones showed a level of care for all aspects of a person. I have heard stories about my grandmother as a midwife in the 1930s–1950s, and about my mother as a physician in the 1980s, that celebrated their willingness to know their patients as people, to help them access resources that weren't just specific to healthcare, and to build meaningful relationships with patients and their families. My journey into music therapy as a form of healing is a direct outcome of the care and service my grandmother and mother lived.

As much as Granny and Mummy attended to the healing of others, they weren't as focused on their own healing. Granny was a very private person and didn't share much with me about her life. To be honest, I was always a little scared of her, especially when it came to our battles over my dislike of oatmeal! She did share about her career but nothing about her personal relationships, struggles, hopes, or dreams. I can only guess that maybe she had experienced some great hurt that made it difficult for her to speak about what mattered to her. My mother was more aware of the need to acknowledge and address things that affected me and my sister emotionally. When she planned to move us to Jamaica, she took us to therapy to process what moving at that stage of our lives would mean and what resources we had to support us. Yet it wasn't until I was well into adulthood that Mummy could speak about her own feelings and struggles. Perhaps Granny and Mummy were operating under the idea that some things aren't for the young people to know; some things are kept close to the vest and never shared. Maybe they didn't know what avenues were available to them to engage in their own healing. Regardless, I know now that healing was important to them, and because of that, my own healing, my own sense of being whole, is a way to honor them and stay connected to them.

In my (Natasha's) own lineage, there was a similar awareness of healing that came from the recognition of how much it was needed or not discussed. There is much I could say about the complicated nature of Afro-Caribbean families, almost all of which I think would resonate with others descended from the Trans-Atlantic Slave Trade. The act of severing Indigenous Africans from their peoples and lands has had a multitude of ripple effects that manifest in today's Black families as complicated histories, family secrets, relationship betrayals, and other ways of, as Resmaa Menakem describes, trauma showing up "as culture."[2] We didn't talk about therapy in our house when I was a child—at least not that I could remember. But we did talk about how the traumas of various past events in our families had shaped us, even if we didn't use words like trauma. As an example, I can recall my paternal grandmother telling me how her father stopped singing after her mother passed away when she was a child. At that time, she urged me to never stop singing, because that expression was important, symbolic of something more than just entertainment, and from that moment I took that urging very seriously.

I grew up in a family of creatives and educators. My mother, who sings and plays the piano, worked in early childhood education, eventually running a clinical training program for undergraduate and graduate early childhood education students. My father, who also sings and plays the harmonica, among several other instruments, taught at the collegiate level in industrial technology, as well as the School of Education, "teaching teachers how to teach." In his retirement, he has taken up a practice of making lovely handcrafted items out of glass and wood. In both my parents' approaches to creativity and education as lifelong learning practices, I see healing as well. There is something I find deeply precious about the experience of watching your parents grow and transform as people, something I realize many of my Ancestors, and even peers, have not gotten to experience. I have seen their parenting practices shift between my own early childhood and that of my younger sisters, heard the words "I love you" increase in use as I aged into adulthood, and I observe them now as playful and tender grandparents. Many of our current familial practices have just as likely stemmed from trauma as from education or creative practice, but the result has been the same (healing), and the creativity and education are the pieces I see as sustaining most strongly. These kinds of stories and experiences are things that I hold as deeply meaningful and critical pieces of myself, and the relationships connected to them deepen with every new practice that emerges. I look forward to continued healing within my family.

We are about to issue another invitation for your own exploration, followed immediately by another, for a total of two. If you're up for it, you can do both back to back or take breaks between them; and remember, these exercises are for *you* first, before anyone else. Think of it as securing your own oxygen mask before trying to assist another person.

Tap in for Reflection: Identify Your Storyholders

Consider: Who are the people, blood-related or not, who hold and share the stories of who "we" are in your family? Write their names in this space:

After you have populated your list, allow your hands to simply sit on the page and—as your comfort/capability allows—read the names slowly, aloud. If that doesn't feel possible for you right now, that's ok! You may consider simply going forward into your week and just paying attention to anything in your environment or history that might draw one or more of these people forward into your mind. Make particular note of anything that happens in your body (tightness/relaxation, any additional urges or emotions, etc.) anytime this happens.

Now let's bring in some creativity!

Pour into Practice: One Storyholder at a Time

When you are ready (as in, when you feel comfortable enough to sit with your list), you are going to choose one of the people or stories that you've identified and find a song to accompany some deeper reflection. Here, we're going to recommend that you go with a person or story that is relatively "low stakes," that is, someone who doesn't stir up feelings that are too deep or strong. They may have been someone who barely made your list, but something in you just knew they had to be there. Song identification is going to be part of how you explore the reason why you knew this. Here are the steps to this process:

1. Write the name/title of the person or story you've selected on a fresh, blank sheet of paper, separate from the list you built previously.

2. Open your platform of choice: you may have a subscription to Apple Music that will make this easier for you. If not, or if you'd rather have videos to work wlth, you can use YouTube.

3. Sit with the name/title you've written, and ask yourself: When I think about this person/story, what sounds, instruments, songs, or artists come to my mind?
    a. If a song comes to your mind right away, hit play!
    b. If a song doesn't come to your mind right away, that's ok! You can google "songs with..." and insert any sounds or instruments that come to mind, or sift through the discography of any artist that comes to mind, to help you gradually narrow down to something that feels right.

4. Take your time! Listen to any songs in their entirety if you can, and don't be afraid to take breaks in this process to let things sit and come back to the list at alternate days/times if need be.

5. As you sit with whatever song you ultimately choose, look at the name/title you've written down and think back to the earlier color/texture exercise, "Pour into Practice: Calculate Your 'Risks and Rewards.'" Is there a color or texture you'd assign to this person/story along with this song? Or anything else that comes to your body/mind that is worth noting?
    a. Document whatever comes up, whether it is a color/texture or other thought or feeling. Even an urge can be noted with a phrase like, "Thinking about this person/story makes me want to..."

6. While you're documenting, resist any urge to build a whole playlist or write beyond a single page at this time—we can do any/all of that later. This is still the time to keep things "small" and allow things to expand from there without pressure.
    a. If you want to save a song to access later, you can "like" it in YouTube or save it to your general library in Apple Music.
    b. If you feel like you want to explore/work through more thoughts/feelings on this story or person, take those thoughts/feelings to someone you trust and start a conversation! If the person/story you thought of is/has a source you can still access easily, maybe you could share the song you chose with them.

7. Breathe through anything that emerges from this experience, without judgment. Check in with your body and meet any needs (hunger, thirst, fatigue) that you may sense, before going on with your day.

There are many directions that a sequence of experiences like this might lead in. You may find you have a deeper sense of clarity or understanding about why the person you chose for the second exercise needed to be on the list you built for the first one. Or you might not. You may feel any number of complex sensations or emotions, or you may feel nothing at all. If you are a helping professional, or someone in a family or community who might benefit from this exercise, you may feel a rushing desire to bring this exercise to someone you work/live with, or you may not. Remember, this time, and this exercise, is about documentation—not judgment! What you are building is a sense of attunement to your body/mind and your intuition, which are critical for recognizing and honoring the influence of your Ancestors on how you think and move today.

In the times before we were able to access someone across the world with a single click, our Ancestors utilized their intuition and creative practice to identify tools and processes for their own safety and well-being and that of those closest to them. These are skills that still have value today, and we honor that Ancestral gift of the opportunity to hone those skills!

Chapter 4

Honoring Our Ancestral Wisdoms

In discussing how each of our lived and historical familial experiences and creative practices has contributed to our personal learnings and development of our own healing practices, we have devised a list of our learnings that we present to you now, with additional context from our emerging understandings of the possible Ancestral sources of these learnings and practices.

Mind, Body, and Spirit Are Integrated

In his pivotal book, *Healing Wisdom of Africa*, Malidoma Patrice Some (who is now an Ancestor) describes an Afro-Indigenous view of healing that integrates mind, body, and spirit.[1] To put it another way, that which affects our mind affects our body, just as that which affects our body affects our spirit, and so on, in an endlessly connected way. This is similar to how the "bodies" or processes of physical and spiritual worlds are connected, as some may be familiar with seeing represented in Kongo Cosmography: the Kongo peoples' way of viewing the world. This is sometimes presented as a diamond or a circle, with four points in the primary colors of red, blue, and yellow, plus black. Many people have conceptualized this imagery in different ways. Natasha has crafted a variation on this Cosmographic image below as a word-based "rune," or a symbol which can be used for meditation or divination, reflecting on the relevant elements noted in each quadrant.

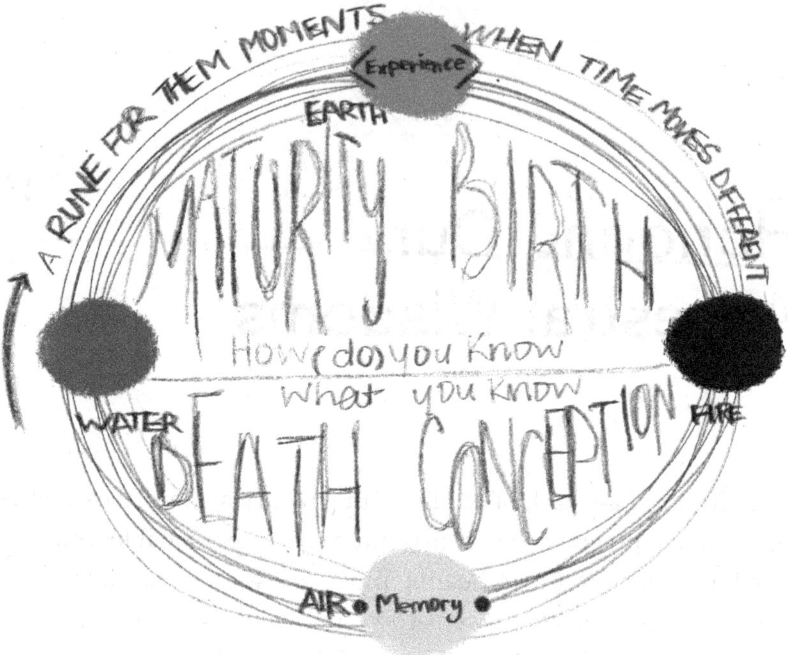

A Rune for Them Moments when Time Moves Different.
A large circle is divided horizontally by a line, framed by the question "How (do) you know what you know." On the left end of the line is the word "Water." On the right end of the line is the word "Fire." At the bottom of the image are the words "Air" and "Memory," and at the top, the words "Earth" and "Experience." Within the circle are the words "Maturity," "Birth," "Conception," and "Death."

The story of how this image evolved is a long and winding one, full of personal insights that aren't critical to the viewing of it but hold great meaning for me (Natasha). What does feel important to share is that while the placement of each element is in alignment with the original Kongo Cosmograph, the flow in which the viewer is encouraged to read the elements is based on my erroneous placement of an arrow that's technically facing the "wrong" direction—my body placed it before my mind could say, "Wait, that's the wrong way!" What's funny is that the original Cosmograph has no arrow at all—arguably, it doesn't need one. Humans experience life as moving from conception to birth, birth to maturity, and then death, so most eyes would probably read the flow of the rune in that order just fine without the aid of an arrow. But my body drew an arrow and pointed it in an opposing direction from the original's flow. So I sat with what meaning I might make from my body's choice, and what I conceptualized immediately affirmed for me that I wanted to leave the "error" exactly where it was, because it reminded me of how that which we experience isn't always all that is influencing any given moment. Sometimes time just "moves different," and things that seem "new" and promising end up being not so sustainable and fade (or die) just as quickly as they appear. When that happens, there's some "growing up" that we have to do (maturity), which can be a humbling experience that makes us feel small and scared, just as birth does. From this place of feeling small, we have to conceive (or remember) new (or Ancestral) ways of being and/or doing in the world, each of which can influence which direction we go next. For me, whenever I can remember and re-integrate the Ancestral parts of myself, then life and time feel more straightforward, moving the "right" way, from conception to birth and maturity, and so on. Still, death is a reality, and so is the experience of getting turned around from time to time. If we were to add another dimension to this circle and make it a sphere, there are even more directions of experience and memory that could be imagined. Thus, this personalized framing of our Ancestor's wisdom is a reminder that, as we've said before, facts aren't everything!

An example of how this Ancestral Wisdom has come up in my (Natasha's) family is through an experience I had with my maternal grandmother in early 2007. Less than a week after her father (my great-grandfather) passed away from cancer at the age of 96, Grandma's spleen ruptured and had to be removed. I happened to be interviewing for a music therapy internship in the area where she lived, so after my immediate family came down to be with her for the surgery, I stayed behind for an extra week after the majority of the family had returned home and supported her recovery. I remember vividly her telling me one day, "My spleen failed because my father died," and that has always stuck with me. At the time, I know that I and other family members in the room at the time kind of chuckled at this, like, "Ok Grandma," but deep down I knew then, and I definitely know now, that she was onto something. Whether or not the breakdown of her spleen was already underway prior to her father's passing, the grief of his loss certainly didn't help her body's ability to function. In fact, what we know of grief and its impact on the body is that it's not at all uncommon for people's immune systems to be compromised during that time; we may not sleep as well or feed ourselves properly, and all that has an impact on our bodies' ability to function.[2] Body, mind, and spirit, all intimately connected, create chain reactions that can ripple into each other and may not be recognizable as connected until they can no longer be ignored.

When I (Adenike) was 16, I had a sort of spiritual crisis. I had great anxiety about the state of my soul and who I was supposed to be. I remember praying a lot but finding little relief. One evening, I felt an intense pain in my stomach. I was doubled over and struggling to eat or drink. As I rarely got sick or complained of anything, my mother was worried and took me to the hospital. The doctor probed and questioned but couldn't figure out what was happening. There was a patient at the other end of the room who was wailing in agony. As I thought about their pain and mine, I grew more afraid and cried out in my spirit for help. I had the sense of being assured that all would be well. Within an hour, I was discharged from the hospital without ever receiving any medication or testing.

Looking back on this incident, I see how I was keenly aware that what was happening to me physically was because of my spiritual and emotional turmoil. I didn't have a way to articulate this to my mother or the doctor, so they were mystified as to what could have been wrong with me. To think this way, of the intertwining of the physical and spiritual, is nothing new. It has always been a part of African cultural worldviews.

In his article about how Yoruba people in Nigeria conceive of health and illness, Ayodele Jegede notes, "the physical and the spiritual are the two dimensions of one and the same universe."[3] What happens in one dimension has an impact on the other. Our Ancestors believed that everything in their daily life from the state of their physical/mental health to the state of their finances, the success of crops to the success of personal relationships, was directly influenced by forces beyond themselves, whether actions of G-d, deities, Ancestors, and/or spirits. As such, it was crucial to perform the necessary rituals and practices that ensured balance between the physical and spiritual dimensions.

Without that balance, their communities wouldn't flourish.[4] To this day, it isn't unusual for Africans across the continent, regardless of their religious affiliations, to go to traditional spiritual healers when facing medical, psychological, and relationship challenges. The comfort, relief, and affirmation that traditional rituals, charms, and divinations offer help people stay connected to their values as they seek to restore balance.

Healing Practice Can Include Spiritual Practice

Recognizing that the mind, body, and spirit are connected presents multidimensional layers of challenges and empowerment. If we know that grief or dreams can have an impact on our physical well-being, then how we tend to those things matters. The way we speak and hold ourselves, the places we direct and hold our attention, all of that has power. I (Natasha) think about how many elders and Ancestors I've heard talk about "speaking into existence," for good or ill. There was a time when I thought of this as a sort of magic switch, like, "I say the thing, and then it happens," but the way I conceptualize it now is more nuanced—that the speaking of an intention, or dwelling on a particular angle of a situation, can be mirrored in our actions, and that can ripple into our health. For instance, if I am constantly expending energy speaking about how much it drains me to spend time with a particular person, I am choosing to continue engaging with them in some way, just by the act of continually speaking about them. What would happen if I changed the frequency with which I referred to them? What peace might find its way into that space? And what other ways might I find to conserve my energy and preserve my peace as a result? On the flip side, if there is something I want to be doing more of, or a person I want to be spending more time with, paying attention to how (and how often) I speak about that aspiration might lead to finding other ways to get closer to it.

Our Ancestors knew this, too. They utilized practices like prayer and engagement with/in physical and communal spaces for that kind of reflection to take place, whether by identifying locations and times of significance in the natural world or through the construction of altars, churches, or other places/opportunities to gather with the people of importance to their lives.[5] These practices run deep and have a ripple effect in and out of our healing as well.

Tap in for Reflection: Assess Your Associations with Spirituality

What happens in your body when you consider the idea of spirituality as being part of a healing practice? Make note of any tension or release that occurs in your body, then allow yourself to briefly consider what might be behind it. Are there messages or stories associated with any of your current sensations? Make shorthand/surface-level notes of those messages or stories as well, not to dive too deeply into them now but just as a temperature check on how this topic lands in your body/mind at this time. Whatever emerges, breathe through it, and remember that beautiful thing about creativity and knowledge: there is always room for nuance, possibility, and difference of perspective between people, and across time!

Considering Altars

The mention of altars can be complex for some people. Another aspect of the legacy of slavery is that it demonized many of our Ancestral spiritual practices. But if we break down the purpose of an altar to its most basic function, as a place for reflection and prayer, many of us have altars in our homes, whether or not we conceive of them as such; they are the bookshelves where we have placed images and keepsakes of our Ancestors, alongside fabric in their favorite colors, or other objects or words they held dear. In my house, my altar space is in my kitchen and includes images of Ancestors, bibles, or tracts that were gifted to me by them, crucifixes, candles, plants, and other objects of significance. When I see them, I feel led to take a deep breath and engage in other practices, like praying, cooking recipes, or singing songs that I learned from them. Your practices may be similar, or different, based on the gifts your Ancestors will have passed on to you.

This also feels like an important place to note that Ancestors do not have to have died at an old age or even be blood relatives. I have Ancestors on my altar who are in no way related to me, and people that passed away at ages younger than I am now. Anyone who has influenced your life in a meaningful way (and that you *want* to remember in a meaningful way, because you don't have to remember anyone you don't want to!), can be an Ancestor. And Ancestors can be remembered with altars, without compromising any other spiritual beliefs. This means, *yes*, venerating your Ancestors and having a relationship with G-d, or your deity/deities of choice, or no deity at all, is all possible! In fact it may all be more connected than you realize. And all of this can be part of your healing process.

That said, remember that every practice/exercise presented in this book is an invitation. You have full autonomy and agency to follow along (or not!) as far as your body/mind feels comfortable. And we mean this! You know yourself best.

Pour into Practice: Tend to an Ancestral Space

Altar tending can be an incredibly nourishing creative and healing practice. As we mentioned, you may already have one or more altar spaces (or something like it, if you'd rather call it/them something else) in your home! Take a moment to think of any space where you have collected images of, or items from, people who were significant to your life and are no longer living. How might you tend to that space today? Perhaps it's something as simple as dusting a picture frame or bookshelf, or picking up a book or other item of significance to that person and holding it in your hands for a moment while you think of them. If you don't have an altar(like) space in your home, perhaps you might build one. Start with just one image or item at a time. Set it somewhere significant, and let time pass as you tend to it, adding or expanding the space only as it feels natural to do so. If the person you are honoring was someone on the list you built in "Pour into Practice: One Storyholder at a Time," maybe you might play the song you identified for them as you build or tend. Natasha actually has a practice of singing songs of personal significance to each of the Ancestors on her altar anytime she tends to that space!

Make note of any sensations or emotions that may arise for you as you take the time to tend to your beloved images or items, without judgment. Meet any bodily or emotional needs that may arise: eat, sleep, cry, or find someone to talk to. Return to this practice, and the documentation of it, periodically to keep it up to date. At this point, there may be emerging evidence of how thoughts/feelings within you may be changing over time. These do not have to be major shifts; in fact, you may not even find yourself shifting in any discernible way other than that you are taking more time to sit with things than you were before. But even that is important, and worth noting!

Keep documenting, as much as you are able. You never know when something might become relevant down the road!

Considering Dreams

As we go deeper into understanding how the physical and the spiritual are connected, we find that the veil between the two realms is thin, and practices in one realm can have impacts in another. One way I (Adenike) experience this is through dreams. It has been said that people dream every night, although most of us don't remember our dreams once we wake up. I know I dream every night and I often remember them upon waking. As a child, I used to wake up every morning and run to my sister saying, "I had a weird dream last night!" and then tell her every detail. My poor sister was so patient with me! This habit of sharing my dreams continued into adulthood, and my sister gave me a journal to record them (I guess that way she didn't have to be bothered with early morning phone calls about my dreams!).

Some of my dreams made sense to me; many didn't. Some of my dreams contained themes, people, and places that I had recently engaged with or was planning to. It wasn't uncommon for me to dream about exams or being late to an interview if I had one of those scheduled the following morning. A few of my dreams felt prophetic. One night in my late teens, I had a dream that I was writing something beautiful and important but I couldn't see the words and I knew that I didn't control the pen. I thought that G-d must be doing that. As I went about my day after waking, I had this strong urge, almost a compulsion, to write a poem of praise and gratitude. I sat down that afternoon and the words just flowed. When I finished, I remembered my dream from the night before and marveled at how my creativity responded to that inspiration.

Other dreams that I've found meaningful have been ones in which I'm spending time with departed relatives. In some of those dreams, my family and I are engaging as though continuing from where we've left off when they lived on earth. Other times, they're aware that they've passed on and have come to share a message with me. In some dreams, the message is symbolic and vague; in others, it is explicit. An example of the latter kind was the second dream I had about my mother after she died. We were standing on the porch of our family home in Trinidad. She looked as I remembered her from my teens—her hair was long and mainly black with a few silver strands, and her face had the barest hint of wrinkles. I was aware that she was preparing to go somewhere and this was my chance to bid her farewell. She said she was going away but that she'd be with my grandmother, great-aunts, and great-uncle who all used to live in our family home. As she spoke, I saw a car stuffed to the gills with things parked at the side of the house. Even though I couldn't see who was inside, I knew that my relatives were in there waiting for Mummy to join them. Mummy told me she'd be fine and I agreed. We parted ways as we used to when one of us was leaving for the day and expected to see each other later. There was no sadness, no sense of finality or loss, but a feeling of assurance that Mummy was going on a good journey to be with family somewhere wonderful.

Dreaming about my Ancestors and receiving messages from them grounds me firmly in the traditions of African beliefs.[6] While there are many communal rituals that invoke the presence, guidance, and blessings of Ancestors, dreams are one way that the individual can receive those things as well. It is possible that when we are in an altered state of consciousness such as a dream state, our minds are less guarded against things we cannot prove with physical evidence. We are more open to our intuition and can receive timeless wisdom that resides in our collective unconscious. We can then use that wisdom to make decisions and take actions that solve problems, that lead us to new opportunities, or that give us hope and peace.

Pour into Practice: "Tune In" to Your Dreamspace

Having a dream is just one more possible step of bridging the physical and the spiritual. Next steps might include remembering the dream and reflecting on the message within it, whether through journaling or speaking with someone about the dream after the fact. Natasha has even utilized a practice in the past of writing short stories based on dreams!

To strengthen your connection to the spiritual through dreams, it might help you to develop specific pre-sleep rituals, like the setting of intentions and avoiding screens for at least 30 minutes prior to sleep. Keeping a dream journal beside your bed will make it easier to record your dreams upon waking, when your memory of them is at its freshest. You could also use the voice memo function of your cell phone or other recording device to recall your dream.

Reviewing what you've written or recorded on your own, shaping it into a short story, or discussing it with someone whose counsel you trust later in the day/week/month might give you insight into what you could do (or need to do!) in response to your dream.

The Spiritual (and by Extension, Healing) is Both Personal and Communal

As personally nourishing as my (Natasha's) spiritual practice is for me, there are extensions of my practice that have ripple effects into my family (and vice versa from them into me as well). As an example, when my maternal grandmother was nearing the end of her life, I asked her to teach me how to make Black Cake, a traditional Caribbean dish usually served around Christmas time. I didn't know anyone else in my family who made it, and even though Grandma had shared her recipe with all of us, I knew how sometimes recipes were only part of a dish, and I wanted to make sure the practice of how Grandma made Black Cake wasn't lost.

I look back on that time of learning from her with such gratitude. Little details like the way she tapped her mixing spoon on the side of the bowl with a little Calypso rhythm, telling me as she did so to study the way the batter dripped from the spoon in order to help gauge the consistency of the cake. It needed to be thick enough to handle the heavy pouring of port wine she would do when it came out of the oven! Another way Grandma told me to test whether the cake was thick enough was to stick the spoon straight up in the batter from time to time and see if it would stay standing—if it did, it was ready for the oven! None of these details would have been found in her written recipe, and I think of her now as I put these practices into my own baking of the cake, which I've done for my family every Christmas now since Grandma's passing in June of 2022. I make the cake, playing music that reminds me of my grandmother and echoing to my children the same reminders Grandma would make to me as I go. Then I pack the cakes with care and ship them to family across the country or bring them with me if I happen to be traveling their way that holiday. This, to me, is sacred practice, and one I know my family looks forward to every year as something that brings us together each Christmas, in remembrance of Grandma.

Some of my (Adenike's) most treasured memories are of the Boxing Day gatherings my mother's family held at my grandmother's and great-aunts' house. Christmas day was usually spent with my immediate family. The day after, we and our uncles, aunts, and cousins would gather at the family home where my grandmother and great-aunts lived. It was the one time each year I was guaranteed to see a large bunch of my extended family outside of funerals. Family members who lived abroad and happened to be in Trinidad for the holidays would also join us. My great-aunt Gloria baked the traditional Christmas dessert of Black Cake. The dining room table wasn't big enough for all of us, so adults would eat in the dining/living room, and the children would take a plate to eat in front of the television or sitting on the porch.

After eating, and the initial shyness had worn off, we'd tell stories and sometimes even sing songs. There'd be laughter, music, and maybe even a steelband passing by on the road.

Looking back, I see how much that was sacred. Our gathering wasn't explicitly religious or spiritual in a ritualistic sort of way, but there was this sense of being together for a purpose. The afternoon and evening were set aside to re-member ourselves amongst those who know and hold our histories. Aunt Gloria didn't only bake our Black Cake, but she would also tell us stories of herself and our grandparents as children. I knew my great-grandmother, Mother Dru, through those stories. Aunt Babsy, Aunt Beryl, Uncle Bernard, and my grandmother would chime in on occasion, confirming or denying what Aunt Gloria shared. My mother and her cousins would also tell newer stories of their youth or stories about my cousins and me that we were too young to recall.

Being with the community of my family helped me to know myself, know my history, and understand where I could go and who I could be. Now that I live far from my homeland and many of my elders have become Ancestors, I am more intentional about being with and in community. I am not fully myself, not whole, if I am not connected and contributing to the people and spaces that align with my purpose and values.

In the summer of 2022, we conducted the first ever BCH retreat. From the moment we agreed to make the retreat a virtual event, one of the first aspects of that retreat that we felt would be important to help ground all of us and bring us together was to have some sort of collective cooking experience. We chose as a dish the Caribbean treat of banana fritters. I (Natasha) used a flexible phone stand to attach my cell phone above my stove as a second camera and then positioned my laptop so my face and upper body could be seen as I walked participants through the mixing of the batter with just three simple ingredients (bananas, sugar, and flour!), just as my own mother had taught me, using some of the same rules about consistency as my maternal grandmother did for Black Cake (when the batter globs onto the spoon and takes a second or two to fall off, then the fritters are ready for frying!). As we cooked together, attendees shared with Adenike and me stories of other comfort foods their families made, and the way those memories and traditions had influenced their lives over time. We bonded collectively as we cooked and then deepened that bond as we ate the treats we had made together. Members of the group posted pictures of their fritters in the group Discord and on social media, some even turning their leftovers into breakfast the next morning, with yogurt or applesauce on top! It was an experience I will always treasure as something that nourished and deepened our time together in a way I don't think we would have found with just a typical, "Hi tell us your name and where you're from," kind of opening.

Tap in for Reflection: Build Your Own Ancestral Wisdoms List

What are your Ancestral Wisdoms around healing? These can be words a family member has said that you hold close whenever you are going through a difficult time, meals that have nourished your soul, or other practices that you have observed being passed down through your family; everything from cold remedies to how you tend to each other during rituals like the birth of a child or death of a loved one is fair game!

Ancestral Wisdoms—a personal list:

Now let's bring in some creativity!

Pour into Practice: Honor Ancestral Wisdom

1. Consider any symbols (images/items, songs, scents, etc.) that come to your mind with any of the stories you've listed above.
2. Doodle your symbol next to the Ancestral Wisdom you associate them with. For instance, if cinnamon is part of a recipe you remember, you might doodle a little cinnamon stick next to that Ancestral Wisdom on your list.
3. Check in with your body and pause to meet any needs that may arise as you do so (for food, rest, etc.).
4. Go on with your day if need be, OR, if you want to take this even further, after you've added your doodles, you might proceed into building a digital or physical collage from magazines or pictures you find online that match (or relate to) what you've doodled, bringing them together in some meaningful way.

Consider as you do so, how might those stories and actions affirm and challenge us to live more fully into our wholeness?

Here is an example, from my (Natasha's) own practice, of the impact that reflecting on Ancestral Wisdoms can have. I call it *The Story of the Many Mothers...*

Once upon a time, I set out to craft a symbolic image for Mother's Day 2022. In a past conversation about family with some other Black Creatives, I had shared images of myself being held by various people, some living, some deceased, and expressed an interest in creating a collage of them. That was where the original idea for crafting this type of image was born: I wanted to create something that merged all these images of me being held, as I strived to hold my own firstborn child, who was four at the time, symbolizing all the love that had always surrounded me my whole life and that I knew would surround them throughout their life as well. I titled that first image "4 mothers holding Momo," which is our firstborn's nickname.

My choice to not include that image here, or the one I created after it, is one of care for the family members to whom I gifted those images. I want to share the learnings from the act of building them, but the images themselves are for my family alone to hold close. That said, I will provide descriptions of the images here, interwoven with the description of the creative and healing process that birthed them, so that the meaning I made may be shared and, perhaps, the healing potential of it may grow within whoever else experiences these descriptions.

In the "4 mothers" collage, an image of me bent forward to hold two-year-old Momo from behind is framed by a combination of flowers and mothers, with a sunset in the background, all excerpted from photos of Momo or myself being held. The photo of my mother, for example, is lifted from an image of her and my dad holding our firstborn, also at the age of two. In the photo behind my mom, her mother holds Momo as an infant. And behind her, my great-grandmother stands with a slight smile, lifted from a photo of her holding me as an infant.

This image was made in a combination of Photoshop and Canva. I Photoshopped the backgrounds out of each individual person's photo and then placed them amidst stock images of flowers and grass from Canva. The image was fun to create, but little did I realize my grandmother would be gone from this earth less than a month later. Then the image became even more precious.

Not long after sharing this gift with my mother, my father expressed an interest in another collage, one that would include the matriarchs of his lineage as well. I was excited by this prospect and sought to collect as many images of these women as possible. I already knew names as far back as five generations beyond myself. Surely there had to be more images out there! So I made some requests for my parents to look, and to ask their siblings to look, and did some digging through my old Ancestry.com folders as well.

Some photos were found, others were not. But I was determined to include all these mothers I knew of, some of whom I'd heard stories about! We just didn't have all the photos.

So, I sat with this determination I felt inside and just started working at trimming the photos I did have and seeing what emerged. By this time, I had started Photoshopping on my iPad instead of my computer. Using an Apple Pencil, I found the process even more enjoyable. It felt more connected, like I was really holding each photo in my hands. I started with an image of my mother, my maternal grandmother, and me, sitting close to each other as I held our firstborn as an infant. That was the original multigenerational photo—before I even had the idea to start collaging images together! As I began nestling that photo against images of my paternal grandmother, and began to frame her photo with images of my maternal great-grandmothers from new (to me) photos I'd received, I began to feel a new and somewhat strange urge to *draw* the mothers I didn't have photos for. I felt this sense that while I might not know exactly what each of these mothers may have looked like, I could at least piece together some aspect of their general shape and try to convey meaning through their bodies based on the stories I'd heard about them. So I started with Ione, the mother of Jewel, my paternal grandmother.

I've told one story of my grandma Jewel here, and for the BCH podcast before; in that story, my grandmother mentions her own mother, specifically in the context that when she died, my grandma's father stopped singing. Grandma was very clear with me that she never wanted me to ever stop singing. And so I asked myself, what kind of woman would make a man sing? I imagined she must have been beautiful. And I imagined she must have been kind, and gentle, as my grandma Jewel was. And so I framed a woman with a heart-shaped face, in similar shades of black and white as my grandmother's photo, one shoulder slightly raised as if she were leaning forward to give her child a goodnight kiss. I found an image of beautifully draped black velvet and used it to craft a sleeve on great-grandma Ione's shoulder. And thus, the rest of the collage began to bloom.

Next to Ione, I placed a dark-skinned woman with a flower in her hair. This was my paternal great-grandmother Margaret, my dad's father's mother. I remember seeing a photo of her long ago, and my dad remembers having seen it somewhere too, but we couldn't find it. I crafted her image here based on what I could remember: that she was dark, and stood with an almost regal posture, and that her hair seemed wavy in the photo, styled in that big-barrel way that so many other Black women of her generation did. I draped her in a navy blue velvet.

Framing my paternal great-grandmothers are my maternal great-grandmothers, Ermine, accompanied by a yellow flower, and Louise, wearing a digitally crafted diamond necklace. I see in Ermine the same sort of mischievousness that my grandmother Dawn possessed. I remember being told she helped care for me as an infant, even though I don't have any memories of her. I wish I did! In Nenny Louise I see a steadfastness and strength that I imagine came from her deep faith. I remember being told that she used to "pray the Psalms" over people, though I can't remember just where that story came from. In each of their stories and faces I feel echoes that I'm certain must have come from their own mothers, and so I crafted Amy behind Ermine and Myrna behind Louise. As your eye progresses from the foreground of the image, where there are more photos, to the background, which is mostly hand drawn, the Ancestors grow larger, such that we only see parts of them, the details getting more and more obscure the further you look. Amy contains the same rosy cheeks as her descendants, a gentle smile spread widely behind that entire first row in the bottom photo! Then we see Myrna's hands, clasped in prayer. Behind Ione, Maude, her mother-in-law (so she would have been my father's grandfather's mother) sings, sunshine pouring from her mouth. Behind Amy, in the far upper left of the corner, an unknown Mother's closed eyes are just barely visible. Through her I pay homage to all the mothers whose names and origins I don't (yet) know.

I hope to continue finding and learning more about all my Ancestors and living my life in a way that continues to honor the many gifts and sacrifices that they gave so that their future generations might have the best opportunities possible available to them. As I crafted this image, Momo would periodically sit beside me, asking, "Who are you drawing?" and "Why?" The story you've just read is an attempt at capturing the things that I told her and the stories I hope to continue passing down to her. I'm pleased to say that when Momo looks at this picture, she can remember which one is Amy, though that may just be because she's the largest figure in the picture (ha!) and her gold-leafed sleeves are so prominently reaching, as if to attempt to hold all of us. Momo's working on remembering the others' names, though. And I hope my children always remain this curious about the many wonderful women who have made the life they live today possible. I also hope they (and you!) feel the same comfort, nourishment, and fortification that I feel imagining my Ancestors behind me at any given moment.

Take a moment to acknowledge each contribution to your own list of Ancestral Wisdoms (including the doodles and any collages you might build!) as a resource, a tool in your toolbox, to be carried forward into your healing journey.

Section Review

In this section, we have discussed Ancestral perspectives on healing and creativity, including:

- the potential for liberation and what's at stake for all of us
- the impact of Ancestors and how to honor them.

We have undertaken the following reflections and practices:

1. Reflect: Describe Sensations, Let Memory Support You
    a. Practice: Calculate Your "Risks and Rewards"
2. Reflect: Describe Sensations (Again!)
3. Reflect: Revisit Your Memories, Risks, and Rewards
4. Reflect: Identify Your Storyholders
    a. Practice: One Storyholder at a Time
5. Reflect: Assess Your Associations with Spirituality
    a. Practice: Tend to an Ancestral Space
    b. Practice: "Tune In" to Your Dreamspace
6. Reflect: Build Your Own Ancestral Wisdoms List
    a. Practice: Honor Ancestral Wisdom

Below is a possible schedule for integrating these practices into your life on a regular basis:

Daily	Weekly	Monthly	As you feel led
Describe sensations: this can be something you do once a day, in the morning or evening, or at multiple points, with as little/much documentation as you feel led!	Tend an Ancestral space	(Re)calculate risks and rewards: what's coming true? What still feels important? Is there anything that needs to be added or removed?	One storyholder at a time: explore more songs, maybe even build a playlist you listen to occasionally. This can also be paired with tending your Ancestral space!
Tune into your Dreamspace by keeping a journal			

Section 2

DIVING INTO THE CURRENT (OF TIME AND POSSIBILITY)

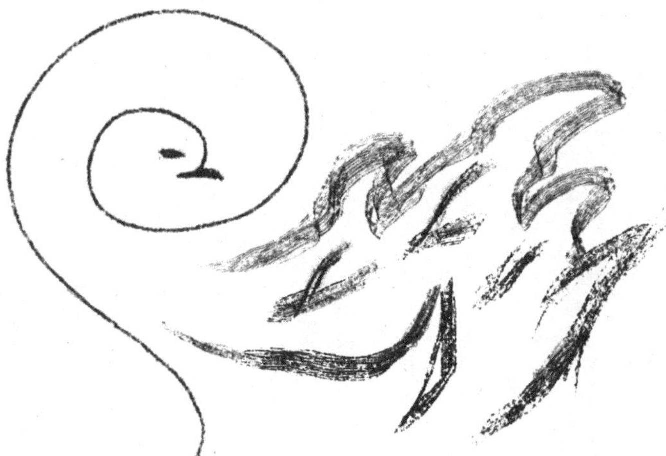

Chapter 5

The Realities of "Healing while Black"

While the Ancestral and liberatory nature of our work renders it accessible to a variety of individuals (not just Black ones!), it feels important to take a moment of intentional re-centering on Blackness in this present moment. The centering of our focus on Black/African Diasporic communities in this work is critical for us, not just because Blackness is our lived experience, but for two additional reasons:

- To quote Taylor Amari Little, "if Africa is indeed the cradle of civilization, then her people are descended from the oldest Indigenous peoples on the planet."[1]
- Also, almost every form of discrimination and oppression in the western world began with the devaluing of the darkest skinned (Black) lives at the intersection of race, gender, and disability, and the impact on us continues to be among the most intense and urgent worldwide.

If we hold both of the above statements as foundational truths, this lends the people of the African Diaspora a certain degree of expertise, particularly those of us walking through the world with the most explicitly visual ties to the Motherland: our skin. We have some of the oldest lived experiences of both indigeneity and oppression. We have arguably seen the fullest spectrum of humanity's wisdom and depravity for the longest extension. If we were to work communally to leverage that knowledge, imagine what the whole of humanity might learn!

Herein lies the challenge: as we've previously stated, there are many sources of knowledge, each of them as unique as the individual possessing them. Part of the challenge of working from such a vast knowledge base is balancing the truth that everyone has knowledge of value while being very specific about your vantage point and the unique way in which it contributes to the tapestry of humanity's history and possibility. To put it another way, this isn't the Oppression Olympics. It's more like trying to help someone find you in a crowd at a location that you are intimately familiar with—that's the kind of expertise we're talking about here. Our perspective matters!

We (Adenike and Natasha) are descendants of Africa, and of the Caribbean. Africa, as a continent, is huge. The Caribbean is very diverse.[2] And so is the United States—and everywhere else you can find descendants of Mother Africa! We have not all had the same experiences, even though the forms of oppression we have faced are all from the same root of colonization. As a result, there is nuance to the many differing strategies we have to survive. This is where it feels important to contextualize our use of the word "Black."

Blackness, particularly in the United States, has served as much as a political delineation as it has a racial category. Malcolm X utilized the term "Black" to apply to anyone non-white, leaning in to the idea that to be Pro-Black was to stand for the capacity of Black people, anywhere, to survive and thrive. In places like the United Kingdom, this is still a standard practice for some, as an effort to highlight the ways in which any deviation from whiteness renders an individual marked as "inferior." When we utilize the term "Black Creative Healing," we are speaking to the experience of "othering," to be sure, and we absolutely position ourselves from a Pro-Black vantage point: we believe in a future with Black people in it and—specifically—a future where all Black people (including our Queer and disabled fam!) are thriving. However, we want to be clear that our use applies specifically to descendants of the African Diaspora living in an explicitly Anti-Black world: that is to say, we live in a world that has been intentionally structured to remind all of us at any given moment that the darker you are, the less opportunity you will have to be seen as "desirable" in any way, and the higher your risk of death. In many ways, we recognize that this framing is deeply—and painfully—connected to the British colonial experience of Blackness that has impacted both of our lives in particular.

Until I (Adenike) moved to the United States, I didn't know I was Black. Let me explain. Growing up in Trinidad and Jamaica, I saw people who looked like me—dark hair, dark eyes, various shades of brown and black skin—in every position and status those societies offered. They owned big and small businesses. They were lawyers, teachers, doctors, nurses, scientists, politicians, and prime ministers. Sometimes people who looked like me were criminals, too. Whenever I entered a public space, I didn't have to justify or prove something because of how I looked and what histories might be associated with that. I did have to make sure not to embarrass my family. Things got around on an island! I saw myself in mirrors and my fellow Trinis or Jamaicans of Chinese, Indian, Lebanese, Syrian, and European descent saw me, but "Black" wasn't necessarily the first thing that crossed our minds. When I came to the United States, and was often the only Black person or person of color in my music classes, I realized that how I look marked me as "different," and that difference wasn't necessarily a desirable or valued thing. Every day I have lived here, I have been explicitly and implicitly made to remember that my race marks me as "less than," alternately someone to be pitied, feared, and ignored, or exoticized and marveled at when I do things not expected of Black people.

But that isn't the whole story of my Black experience. Being Black in the Caribbean has its own generational wounds to address due to how slavery and colonialism happened. That was something I had already had to unpack for myself. Immigrating to the United States and being faced with Anti-Blackness rooted in a similar yet different tale of slavery and colonialism adds a layer of complexity to my efforts to engage in my healing. In many ways, I do not experience the full brunt of Anti-Blackness that Black/African-Americans have endured since birth. Frequently, when non-Black people hear my accent and learn of my place of birth, they are intrigued, curious, and friendlier than they were when they first saw me. For the first half of my life in the United States, I took that to mean I was exceptional and perhaps better than Black people born here. It took years for me to recognize and begin to unlearn the Anti-Blackness that I had internalized, a lot of that as a result of consuming biased media depictions of Blackness when I lived in the Caribbean. With increased reports of instances of police brutality against Black people, with statistics that show Black people continue to earn less and have fewer material resources than their white counterparts, along with everyday instances of covert discrimination and harm, I have learned over the years that I am no different, no better or worse, than my American Black siblings. Non-Black people will see my skin color first and make a decision about their actions towards me based on that.

I (Natasha) was raised by parents who similarly "discovered" that they were Black upon arrival in the United States. As such, I remember being told at a very young age that I was going to be held to a different standard than my peers. As with many children of immigrants, this then evolved into languaging and practices that promoted a line of thought that I had to be smarter, better dressed, more polite, etc. as a default, when compared with my non-Black peers, because I was not going to be given the benefit of the doubt that my white counterparts would be. And while there was truth in that framing, it also lent itself to my own internalization of Anti-Black thought. I looked down on other Black folks who didn't appear to be "trying" as hard as I was. I began to see myself as some sort of "better other," when the reality of Anti-Blackness is that it doesn't matter how much money you appear to have or how educated you are: at the end of the day, if you're Black, that's all some people are ever going to see of you. And that realization can be devastating.

This is why contextualization of our perspectives and vocabularies is important. Because Anti-Blackness would have us fracture ourselves and fight each other in an effort to fit into spaces that simply were never designed for us. We call these the "Diaspora Wars" and they are very real! Folks from Africa arguing with folks from the Caribbean about what is the "right" way to pronounce, or do, or be, this thing or that thing. None of those fights ever get us anywhere. As Ancestor Toni Morrison has said, "the very real function of Racism is distraction."[3] And Anti-Blackness is very good at distracting us from the reality of our (Black folks') situation, which is actually quite dire if you think of it. All over the world our life expectancy and general quality of life is significantly lower than our non-Black counterparts. We are dying earlier and with fewer of our dreams fulfilled. Fighting each other will not help this.

This isn't to say that we can't enter into discussion about the ways in which we view or experience the world differently from each other—we can, and we should! What we do want to be clear about (re)stating, here, is that we do not believe anyone ever deserves to be harmed, so lashing out at each other isn't cool, and you're allowed to distance yourself from people and/or spaces where you do not feel safe or affirmed.

What we are speaking to here is the value—in spaces where we feel safe and affirmed—of recognizing points of fracture and being able to say, "Here is where I have come from and what I have seen, tell me what you have seen" (and then listening to the responses and empowering each other to move interdependently from our unique vantage points!). We believe that the more of us can do this, the more of these oppressive systems we will be able to see and dismantle more thoroughly.

We'll speak more about the idea of interdependence, and the beautiful potentials therein, in the coming chapters. Until then, we honor the Black British framing of Political Blackness, and the framing of Black American thinkers like Malcolm X that help give voice and purpose to our Pro-Black aspirations, and we recognize that the language we use is also unique to our lived experiences as African Diasporic Descendants living in the United States, and that the experiences of our readers may vary.

Tap in for Reflection: Define Your Connection to Africa

Check in with your body for a moment: how are you feeling as you read all this? Is there tension anywhere that you might need to release? How's your breath? Your hunger or energy levels? Maybe take in some extra oxygen, feed yourself, or drink some water as you read the following poetic affirmation:

"I see Africa in you, and I honor it.
Whether it is blood that runs through your veins,

or blood that your Ancestors have touched.
I call it Mother.
Tell me where your Ancestors come from.
Here is the African in me: she is old, gray,
full of wisdom and wit.
And pain too.
All of life has been her teacher.
What might we learn from each other?
What meaning might we make from this Blood of the Mother?"

Take a deep breath.

Now take another.

Now... let's bring in some creativity!

Pour into Practice: Breathe into Your Connection(s)

This is going to be our first official invitation to use your body, beyond writing something down or taking a deep breath. You are going to develop a small movement or gesture. We recognize that moving our bodies may feel strange or uncomfortable for some people, so we are going to intentionally keep this small, and again, remember, you are in control! If something feels like it pushes beyond the realm of reasonable discomfort for you, stop and reset. There is time, and there are many paths we might take. Work with what works for you.

1. Ask yourself: What is my **connection** to the African continent? In what way(s) does that connection manifest?
   a. Maybe it is blood, as the poem above mentions, or maybe you know a story of your family that connects you in history, or maybe the connection is just the world we live in now and the Black folks who occupy the spaces in which you live and work.
   b. Take a moment to just sit with your answer.

2. Now ask yourself: If I were to **imagine** that connection as something **tangible**, what would it be? A piece of string? A strand in a web? A wave in the ocean? Where in my body does that string/strand/wave connect? And what does that feel like?
   a. The question of how something "feels" may lead you into an intellectual answer: resist this! You want to feel into your body in a literal way. This may mean bringing one or both of your hands to a point in your body where a string/strand/wave might touch you and imagining the sensation of such an object/texture.
   b. Breathe into the feeling.

3. When you feel as though you have a grasp of how your connection to Africa feels in your body, take a deep breath, and as you exhale, let your body *make some small movement or gesture—just for a moment!—in a physical response to that connection.*
   a. This is your Connection Gesture, and it could be as small as the breath itself, or you may need to take a second or third breath before a movement comes. Let instinct guide you!
      i. Examples: If you've conceptualized a string or a strand, maybe your hands grasp that string/strand and pull, ever so slightly. Or if you've imagined a wave, your body might rock forward and backward slightly.
   b. Whatever it is, if you feel comfortable with this small movement, repeat it a few times. If not, just let the movement moment pass and breathe into stillness afterwards.
   c. Take note of how the feeling of engaging with that connecting sensation might settle or move through your body or emotions.

4. Meet any needs that might arise from this point, including creative needs! If you are a natural mover or a dancer, go

ahead and put on a piece of music (maybe even the piece you chose earlier in "Pour into Practice: One Storyholder at a Time" to represent a person/story in your family!) and let your body move even further. Or maybe you need to show this movement to someone else. Or maybe none of this applies to you, and you just need to think about all this for a while before you can move forward into your day or whatever comes next. It's all possible, and only you know what's best for you.

5. Breathe.

Chapter 6

The Thing about Western Medicine

As we contextualize our own experience of Blackness in the global landscape, we also need to contextualize African Diasporic perspectives on healing amidst the backdrop of dominant western (white/Eurocentric, Christian, heteronormative, patriarchal, and ableist) practices. These are the foundational beliefs and practices that shape the environments in which many of us have been raised and indoctrinated.

The practice of western medicine has long been regarded as the pinnacle of scientific achievement and professional prestige. With the technological advances and biomedical research that have occurred in the last 150 years, we seem to have gotten closer to unlocking all the secrets of the body and of controlling what it does. The arc of the story seems to suggest that humans really are the lords of all—the world around them and the realms within them. Yet, new viruses emerge that threaten global shutdown. There is still uncertainty about how many psychiatric medications actually work and what implications they have for overall health. And so humans continue to seek knowledge and mechanisms to eradicate viruses, fix "defective" systems and organs, and control the quantity and perhaps quality of life we get to live. This idea of control, mastery, or dominance is also what guided the spread of colonization by various western/European countries. Other lands, peoples, and customs were to be brought under western/European control or eradicated. In much the same way, the values, principles, and practices of modern medicine can be considered to be colonizing the values, principles, and practices of non-western/non-European cultures.

If we compare the prevailing values underlying health/healing practices in many African cultures with those centered in conventional western medicine, we will find reflections of fundamentally distinct understandings about life.

Compartmentalization of Body, Mind, and Spirit

In the last few years, I (Adenike) have had more doctors' visits than usual. I experience a strange symptom or pain, so I make an appointment to see my primary care physician. She may refer me to a specialist like a neurologist to better determine what's going on and how to treat it. I also have regular checkups with my gynecologist and some visits with a counselor. All of the clinicians I see focus on a specific aspect of my well-being and functioning. They could all belong to the same healthcare network and have access to my medical record containing my history and current medications, but still, they only focus on what pertains to their specialty and what they deem pertinent to their realm of expertise. Even within a physician's office there can be a lack of communication and integration. On one visit to my gynecologist, my blood pressure reading was particularly high when the nurse took it. When the doctor came in, we discussed my history since the last visit, and she was about to write me a new prescription for birth control when I commented on my blood pressure. Upon hearing what the reading was, she said that we had to go in a completely different direction with my options for birth control. I was taken aback by the thought that not only had the doctor not read the information that the nurse wrote in my chart but that if I hadn't said something, she would have prescribed me medication that could have made me experience some serious complications.

In my experience of western medicine, I am an assortment of distinct needs and concerns. Very rarely do I experience being seen as a whole person comprised of integrated domains. My primary care physician never asks about my spiritual life as part of understanding my experience of my physical symptoms. I am grateful that there are specialists who have spent a lot of time studying and working with particular systems and organs of the body. It's helpful and a huge relief to go to a physician and get targeted help for specific concerns. Yet it is frustrating to spend months or even years trying to address a concern by going to multiple specialists, often working in silos, when the solution might require a more integrative, wholistic approach.

Much of my (Natasha's) young adult life was spent trying to figure out the source of mysterious and constant pain. It started (or so I thought at the time) in my hands and was frequently accompanied by widespread aches and intense physical fatigue. My doctors at that time considered rheumatoid arthritis, lupus, and multiple other conditions before finally landing on fibromyalgia. But in time, other symptoms appeared, and my diagnoses got more complex. Maybe it wasn't fibromyalgia, or maybe it was fibromyalgia and something else? Later in my 20s, when my spouse and I started trying to conceive and weren't having any success, I spent a lot of time in OB-GYN offices and found out that I had PCOS (polycystic ovary syndrome) and endometriosis. I remember one doctor telling me that when they looked at my chart as far back as my teen years, they could see the signs. Another one told me that the nausea I described getting during "that time of the month" might actually have been a pain response but that the pain was just so intense that my body could only register it as vomit-inducing. Even my fatigue and broader experiences of pain began to make more sense. My flares weren't random. They were part of a specific network of hormones and tissues going haywire.

Hearing this at a time when I was also beginning to think more wholistically about my life in general was foundation-shifting. I began to ask myself, what else do I experience in my body at particular times in my menstrual cycles that might actually be more tied to that part of my body than anything else? I began obsessively charting everything from my body temperature upon first waking every morning to pain levels and how I was feeling emotionally by the end of each day. And I learned a *lot*. But let me be clear: that level of charting is not for everyone! What I uncovered wasn't exactly great for my mental health. While I figured out many connections between symptoms, some things (like the very specific pain in my hands) still didn't make sense, and

I began to experience all new cycles of self-blame and shame for not "catching" the connections that did exist earlier, and beating myself up for not being able to figure out what connections I might be missing. Knowing what I know now, though, I can't imagine my health journey unfolding any other way, given the hyper-individualized and compartmentalized system in which we live.

Individual Responsibility vs. Care in the Context of Community

In modern western medicine, the physician engages with the patient not just within their specific scope of training but solely as an individual. The symptoms and conditions a patient has are often initially understood solely in the context of that patient. Someone's good health is their responsibility, and if they have an illness or disease, it is probably due to their actions or inaction. This way of viewing health reflects the individualism that is a key element of the western/European worldview. Everything starts and ends with the individual; their success or failure at life is solely based on their efforts. While in some ways this mindset celebrates human potential and encourages striving for excellence, it completely dismisses the role and impact of inequity, oppression, and discrimination in the lives of minoritized individuals. It also places pressure on individuals to achieve unrealistic standards, as it ignores the presence and function of interdependence and collective engagement. When using this worldview to design healthcare, physicians and other clinicians miss out on big pieces of the picture. Their understanding of a patient in front of them is limited at best and could be lethal at its worst.

It wasn't until more recently, like within the last 30 years, that western physicians began to consider social determinants of health (i.e., family, social, and socioeconomic factors) when assessing a patient's needs and well-being.[1] Where and how someone lives and works and the level of access they have to health resources directly affects their well-being. This tells us that policy decisions and the actions of those controlling resources can contribute to the presence of "good health" or "ill health" in a community. Yes, an individual is responsible for choices they make in terms of how they nourish and care for their body; however, if their neighborhood is designed in such a way that there are more fast-food restaurants than any grocery stores selling fresh produce and other "healthy" food options within a reasonable distance, no recreational spaces for exercising, and limited job opportunities that would pay a living wage to allow someone to afford more than just the dollar menu at McDonald's, then it is almost impossible for them to consistently be well.

Social determinants of health are not the only aspects of community factors that influence health. The values, beliefs, attitudes, and practices of various cultural groups also directly affect how someone experiences health and well-being. Many non-western/non-European cultures have a collective worldview which places the individual within the context of something bigger than themselves. In those cultures, an individual understands who they are and how they show up in the world through interacting with their family, and social and other communal groups. The strength and frequency of interactions with others can determine whether an individual sees themselves as being well or unwell. Social well-being influences emotional well-being, which can show up in the presence or absence of physical symptoms.

Zambian music therapist Nsamu Moonga also describes the ways that Indigenous communities have historically responded to the presence of unwell-ness in their midst as being communal.[2] One person's wellness is the community's wellness, so anything that compromises the individual is the community's responsibility as well. People may gather to share resources or enter into ritual together. Everyone has a role to play, and everyone has value. This is affirmed over and over again by the community's responses to individual needs. Research also tells us, however, that if you place those same people into a context that does not value their collective understandings of the world, those same people will actually experience *more* distress, even though their viewpoints have not changed.[3] Their isolation becomes a negatively contributing factor.

For me (Natasha), I was raised in an environment that frequently downplayed pain. Whether emotional or physical, the intersection of the British colonial upbringing of my parents and the highly conservative upper Midwest in which my identity was forged led to a strong internalization of having a "stiff upper lip," or learning to "grin and bear it," with regards to pain. This is not something I consider to be any one individual's fault—it was simply an impact of the systems in which we were all embedded. I witnessed members of my family and community demonstrating this "downplaying" behavior, and heard it revered as a virtue, a strength. As a result, I remember feeling like, as a kid, I had to either hide any pain I was experiencing as long as possible, or—if I couldn't do that, become very loud about it in order to be heard. But even that didn't always work, because then I began to be viewed as somewhat of a hypochondriac. And then, even *I* began to believe that I couldn't really be experiencing what I was experiencing, because it was all in my head, wasn't it?

It wasn't until I began to see and hear of other people experiencing similar types and combinations of pain as myself that I began to make more connections between what I was feeling and what might be the cause of it. For instance, I now know that the pain I experience in my hands comes from the intense picking of the skin around my fingers that I engage in as a form of self-stimulation (stimming), most often when I am stressed.[4] The positions my hands form to do this are often claw-like, and the impact of this during stressful periods, where I'm also using my hands to type or play an instrument, is cumulative. I've had two surgeries for carpal tunnel syndrome and had never once considered that the origins of my pain were due to this neurological urge to stim, which is brought on by my ADHD (attention deficit hyperactivity disorder). This is a diagnosis I didn't receive until I was in my 30s, partially because my symptoms were largely "manageable" until they weren't (fun fact: hormones—like those produced when you have a baby—can influence ADHD!). My diagnosis was also complicated because of the way ADHD manifests in girls socially, particularly Black girls. The way western society impacts our development is not part of the general public's awareness of how ADHD exists. We are often just coded as being "overemotional" and subconsciously conditioned to hide or mask our symptoms by turning our stimulation needs into our bodies with actions like skin picking or hair twirling, because it's not "ladylike" for us to work out our hyperactive urges in the ways more stereotypically coded male counterparts do. I know this now because of conversations I have had with other ADHD-ers (particularly Black ones) who were able to point me towards the resources I needed to get my diagnosis and treatment—treatment that has truly changed my life. I have less physical pain now than I used to because I can catch the signs of stress earlier than I could before, and all because I began to have conversations (and develop community!) with people who were living with similar experiences to my own. This is something my Ancestors, and Indigenous people around the world, have known generationally, despite the efforts of western/individualistic notions of health. I just had to find my way back to it.

Community building/re-integration, through conversations and other connections, has the power to break the shame cycles we can become stuck in and lead us towards deepening relationships with people and practices that can help us tremendously. I think about the Dysautonomia International Black Support Group that I have found on Facebook, or the neuroexpansive spaces I've become connected to via Instagram. Some of these have been thanks to Google searches, and others have come from me just being more vocal about my experiences and recognizing connections within my existing social connections. Conversations and connections in a system as deeply racist and ableist as ours, can literally change lives.

Tap in for Reflection: Contextualize Your Experience of Pain

Who in your life do you talk to about pain (whether physical, emotional, or otherwise), other than doctors or related health professionals? Where do those conversations happen? And how do you talk about pain with those people/in those spaces? Begin to make note of the descriptive adjectives you use to describe your pain. Below is an example from Natasha. Your own table might look similar, or different.

Who I talk to about pain	*Where* those conversations happen	*How* I describe my pain
Example: My spouse/ family **My experience:**	Example: At home, in phone (audio/video/text) communications **My experience:**	Example: Cramping, tightness, draining **My experience:**

Now let's bring in some creativity!

Pour into Practice: Poetic (Re)Construction

Look at your list of how you describe pain. Read it like a poem. As you do so, allow yourself to take some creative liberties—maybe move a punctuation mark around or move some words onto a new line. As you make each change, pause and sit with what you're creating, looking at the words like they're a piece of visual art. Do they look the way you want them to?

Allow yourself to play with even the most fundamental "rules" of grammar or spelling. You have that power! And as you do this, ask yourself: What other power might I have? What else might I be able to shift, in even the smallest of ways?

I (Natasha) think of how a therapist of mine once encouraged me to visualize a volume knob on my pain or that I had a remote in my hand that could "turn the volume down," even slightly. That practice has proven to be incredibly effective for me, particularly on days where my pain level might feel impossible to manage. Even at its worst, I can always turn the volume down a notch or two, and even that small action can grant me critical breathing room to go on with my day with just a little more sense of presence and clarity, and not just for myself! When I am able to breathe a little easier and move a little more freely, this has an impact on my relationships as well, which then feed back into me as I feed into them, in a never-ending cycle.

Beyond the role of interpersonal relationships in individual health needs moment to moment, the communal healing practices of non-western/non-European cultures can also determine how an individual experiences well-being overall through consistent community practice.[5] For instance, among some Indigenous/Native American (also called American Indian) communities, a sweat lodge is a communal practice that is believed to remove impurities from the body while renewing the spirit, and community members are encouraged to engage with this practice on a regular basis, whether or not they feel a specific need in the moment. Regular engagement in these communal practices help members of these communities feel well and whole more consistently and sustainably. Sometimes practitioners of western/European medicine underestimate the value of such practices or even condemn them as unhealthy. Whatever may be believed about the physical impact of the sweat lodge, think about the conversations that may happen in that kind of communal space, or others similar to it, like a sauna or the pedicure station of a salon. There can be a sense of community forged by common experience. And that can be healing in and of itself! But if western/European medical practitioners only promote and prescribe those "healthy" remedies that they know and value, they run the risk of causing harm to an individual's well-being by disconnecting them from a core aspect of their identity and cultural practices, which are often where the more felt senses live, and where meaning is made. All this can have major impacts on the health of a person's body, mind, and/or spirit (which, as we've discussed previously, our Ancestors knew to all be connected!).

Minimization of the Role of Spirituality in Health

When I (Adenike) first began my music therapy training in the latter part of the 1990s, we didn't talk much about spirituality and the role it plays in someone's well-being. There was this sense that I should never bring up spirituality unless the person I was working with did, and even then, it was a topic to skirt around. Back then, my understanding of spirituality was tying it to a specific religion, and since music therapy wasn't a religious practice, spiritual goals were not things to consider. It wasn't that my instructors didn't acknowledge the role of spirituality in people's lives; rather, it was more about having students understand and stay within a scope of practice. As I started my first job working with older adults, spirituality became something I had to reckon with. Was it fine to play hymns one person requested if another person in the group wasn't Christian? Was it ok to pray with someone if they felt inspired to do so after our music-making? If I made things easier for myself by avoiding all references to spiritual things, would that be a problem for the people I worked with?

The tension I felt with these questions emerged as a result of the compartmentalized approach prevalent in western/European healthcare. Medicine seemed to preoccupy itself with the study and treatment of what is empirically observable. How does one empirically observe, quantify, and study the spirit? In the latter part of the 20th century, there was increased interest in acknowledging and understanding connections between physical well-being and spiritual well-being. Researchers found that patients who engaged in a spiritual or religious practice tended to report increased quality of life and some reduction in pain.[6] There is more intentionality with understanding a patient's relationship to their spirituality and having chaplain services and other pastoral care resources available in hospitals. As welcome as this is, there is still a sense of spirituality being an extracurricular in the program of life and not a core subject.

In contrast, as we talked about earlier, many African cultures have a worldview in which spirituality is integral to how life functions and is organized. It is not uncommon for African patients to pursue spiritual remedies for physical ailments before or in addition to conventional western/European medical care. Each person is an integration of spirit and physical matter; both are equally important in understanding what it is to be alive and to be a person. For members of the African Diaspora and their descendants, solely relying on the worldview that western/

European medicine employs denies their full personhood and invalidates a significant aspect of their lived experience.

One of my (Natasha's) current research projects involves studying the relationship between music and stress in Black families of children with sickle cell disease (SCD), which predominantly impacts descendants of the African Diaspora. While the details of that study have been published elsewhere, I can share personally here that the experience of working on that study has amplified for me how connected so many of our Black/African Diasporic families' spiritual practices are to our sense of emotional and physical well-being.[7] Having a practice of going to church (whether your church is a physical religious structure or simply spending time in nature, which is what my father likes to call his church!), taking your concerns "to church" or leaving something "on the altar"/"in God's hands" via the act of prayer can have a tremendous impact on a person's stress level, which in conditions like SCD (or neurodivergences like ADHD) can be critical to that person's overall quality of life.

Tap in for Reflection: Stories of the Inexplicable in Health

Many individuals have family stories of seemingly impossible occurrences in their family's health history. Some may call these miracles, while others simply acknowledge them as "luck" or synchronicity. These may be stories that you've been encouraged to hide in the past, or only tell to certain people, like someone coming back from the brink of death, or opening their eyes in the moment before departure from life, right after hearing a prayer or song that held meaning for them. Sometimes these moments are among our most precious memories. Take some time to document one such story from your family. As you do, take note of what happens in your body/mind, and meet any needs that may arise—to feed yourself, rest, or reach out to a loved one—before moving on to the rest of this chapter.

Curative vs. Preventive/Context-Based Approaches

Typically, those of us living in places where western/European medicine is the predominant mode of healthcare seek out a doctor or other health clinician when we experience something in our bodies as not functioning like we think it should. It's possible that we wait until we don't feel well to think about healthcare, because the prevailing attitude in western/European medicine seems to be one of fixing something after the fact. It's also possible that due to lack of access to resources for affordable healthcare, we tend to seek care when things get really bad. In the United States, the passing of the Affordable Care Act in 2010 sought to make it easier for people to access healthcare as well as to pursue preventive or more context-based health measures.[8] [9] These measures allow patients and healthcare providers to consider where care recipients live, their social determinants of health, and what needs may accompany their unique position in the world and merit focused attention. Granted, a shift to more explicitly address preventive and context-based measures may have initially been driven by a comparison of the financial costs involved in treating things like cardiac arrests and diabetes with the costs of supporting people in being more educated about those things. Even with this shift, however, things still skew more on the curing and reactive side than the preventive and proactive contextual side.

This isn't to say that there haven't ever been curative approaches used in Afro-Indigenous communities. Many African cultures have incorporated spiritual practices that honor Ancestors and deities for curative purposes, alongside practices meant to prevent misfortune. This is rooted in a belief that by maintaining certain community and spiritual traditions, people could stave off or avoid many difficult situations. Historically and continuing today, members of various African communities seek natural and spiritual remedies rooted in our awareness of the land, our plant relatives, and the many gifts of the recipes our Ancestors curated over time to help us live more comfortably and wholly.

All that said, Ancestral practice can sometimes be like a game of telephone. As our Ancestors developed their tools amidst unbelievable trauma, they were also developing coping mechanisms and ways of perceiving, being, and doing in the world that served specific protective purposes that were time-bound to the situations in which they were living. When we can be mindful of this context, we can also become aware of how some of our Ancestral understandings may not be applicable in every context or may have become distorted as each generation has passed it down. The results of these kinds of misunderstandings or mis-applications can be seen in those of us who would seek to treat symptoms of "ill health" with a hyper-focus on "high vibrations" and/or other aspirational goals that can be counter to the process of actually healing in all your wholeness. We have to be careful of curating our own shame spirals out of Ancestral Wisdoms. Our Ancestors lived when they lived and did the best they could with the tools they had at the time. Those of us who are alive now have information and tools that they didn't have in their time, so it's important to stay grounded (and humble!) in both our current and Ancestral contexts.

Think of yourself as part of a deeply interwoven tapestry that is also a sort of formula or code that can be updated over time. Each strand or thread of code is unique from every other thread that surrounds you, with new threads being added every day! As such, it is impossible to be separated from any other thread without having an impact on the whole. Be mindful of that which could cause you damage, just as you are mindful of that which would cause harm to anyone else.

With this in mind, because healing is an ongoing process, and not necessarily a finite one, the most effective Ancestral practices do not aim to bury or destroy any mere presence of illness, "lowness," or pain; instead, they recognize it as part of the human experience, something to be acknowledged, faced, recognized, and integrated as part of us, not as detracting from who we are. Having a balanced and contextual awareness of times, uses, and other critical contexts around curative and preventive approaches for health reflects a wholistic, integrative approach to sustaining individual and communal well-being. Discernment is part of how we get there.

Pour into Practice: Attune to Your Sense of Bodily Knowing

We're jumping straight to the art on this one!

You're going to be trying an adaptation of "Somatic Self-Portraits," a Creative Body-Scanning exercise that I (Natasha) first had the gift of experiencing from Ellen Bartel during a conference gathering of the International Somatic Movement Education and Therapy Association (ISMETA). This is what you will need:

- Your body, fed and well rested, or as close to those as you can get it!
- A piece of paper.
  - Any kind will do, but if you want to spring for cardstock or something with similar thickness, that might be beneficial.
- Something to write/draw with.
  - Ideally this will be a tool that won't bleed through the paper or struggle with an uneven surface (because you won't be working with a table or anything super firm to press on!). I recommend a gel pen or a non-mechanical pencil.
  - If you have thicker paper, a marker would probably be fine, and may in fact yield the clearest results!
- Time: at least ten minutes.
  - You can set a timer for the first five minutes or listen to a song of that length while you work.

Please note that this is an exercise that is going to invite you to "scan" your body with your mind's eye, from top to bottom, and then move your hand/tool with this scan in mind. This is something that people may have varying degrees of challenge or comfort with. Remember, only you know your limits, when you are in a space to be challenged, and when a challenge might actually be unsafe for you to engage with. Move forward only at the pace of your own capacity, with care.

Here's exactly what you'll be doing with those tools:

1. Hold the paper up to your chest with one hand and your tool in the other.
   a. Let whatever hand is holding the paper be in contact with both the paper and your body.
   b. Let whichever hand is holding your tool rest gently on your lap for now.

2. Breathe. Feel the paper and your hand rising and falling, in time.

3. Close your eyes. Let your mind center in on the top of your head, imagining a sensor just above it, gently collecting data.
   a. You are in charge of that sensor, its movement, and how much data it collects.

4. When you're ready, imagine that sensor moving downward from the top of your head to the tips of your toes. As it moves, bring your tool hand up and place the tip of the tool to the paper. Keep your eyes closed. The idea here is to let your hand move in response to your whole body and not be influenced by your visual perception of whatever emerges.

5. On your next exhale, begin to move the tool to draw a representation of your body from top to bottom, as perceived by the sensor you are controlling, in response to the signals that sensor is giving you.
   a. An example of this can be found in this TikTok video I recorded of myself doing this exercise in 2021:

www.tiktok.com/@blackcreativehealing/video/6937759473989717253

b. Your drawing will not be literal in any sort of "photorealistic" way. Resist the urge to be "certain" of whether what you're drawing looks anatomically correct or aesthetically pleasing. Whether the thing "makes sense" in a visual way is not the point. You are responding to sensations in your body first. You can look later.
    i. Example: Feeling tension anywhere? Breathe, notice it, then let your tool hand move in whatever way that sensation has motivated your hand to!
    ii. Moving in response to your body's sensations may result in tapping or dragging your tool against/across the paper on your chest in patterns that may or may not resemble anything visually, and that's ok. Just work your way through your body, and the paper, from top to bottom, interpreting each sensation with your tool.

6. When you have reached the bottom of your body, or your paper (whichever happens first), stop. Breathe. Thank your body for the messages you are about to interpret.

7. When you are ready, turn your paper around and look at it.
    a. What do you feel when you look at it?
    b. How would you describe what you see and what you feel in response, i.e., when you look at a certain marking you made with your tool, can you tell what sensation you were responding to?
    c. If you feel so led, write your description(s) down (so you can reference them later!).
    d. Now: take a moment to explore what might be in between what you see and how you feel. This might be through more writing, finding additional words to flesh your descriptions out, or leveraging your body in a way similar to the exercise "Tap in for Reflection:

Define Your Connection to Africa," letting movement be your tool for interpretation for those bits of connective tissue between your feelings and thoughts.

e. You may not feel led to do anything more than sit with what you feel when you look at the paper—and that's ok too! In the coming sections, we're going to go deeper with our creative choices and actions, but this is one last moment to just sit with the top layer of what you are sensing and experiencing.

8. Save your portrait somewhere safe (because we may return to it later!) and go on with your day, with gentle attention to your body's needs—keep it as hydrated/fed/rested as possible!

Glorification of Pharmacology over Natural Remedies

In many societies that rely on western/European medicine, a lot of attention is placed on using drugs to address health needs. Thanks to advances in science and technology, researchers have identified and created compounds that can interact with and control processes and organ functions in our bodies. Medical practitioners place significant value on pharmacologically-derived drugs based on evidence that supports their effectiveness and reliability. For many people, these drugs are welcome inventions that save their lives. Yet there are often severe side effects, known and unknown, that make pharmacology something to be dealt with cautiously. Again, a place for discernment.

Another aspect of concern, especially in the United States, is the cost of these drugs. Without insurance (and sometimes even with it), many of these necessary drugs are unattainable, as they are extremely expensive. It's not uncommon for pharmacists and other healthcare professionals to tell stories about patients who have to choose between buying food and paying bills or buying their medications. Being well, as understood within the western/European medical industry, is directly tied to socioeconomic status and access to resources. Those with minimal or no access to well-paying jobs that provide insurance, alternatively affordable options for insurance, affordable clinics, or money to cover basic needs barely get a chance to be well in all senses of the word. Turning to natural remedies might be a game changer, as they may be more readily available to folks with few resources.

Our African Ancestors and many of our siblings within the Diaspora frequently rely on natural remedies to promote well-being and treat ailments. This trust in naturally growing and obtainable solutions reflects the perspective of being connected to one's environment and other forms of life. We are in relationship with our environment, and through that relationship, we know ourselves and we know what it is to be well. To say that continued reliance on natural remedies is sentimental or unquestioning adherence to outdated traditions is to dismiss a key understanding of the worldview of many African cultures. Those remedies weren't just relevant in times when technology was not advanced or resources were scarce. Those remedies are tangible ways of reinforcing the understanding that we are connected to all that is around us; there is no distinction between the energy in me and the energy in the earth. Relying on the earth's resources to sustain our well-being reminds us that we are in a reciprocal relationship with our environment—we take turns caring for each other.

Even within modern societies that prioritize western/European medical approaches, you can still find folks with ties to various Indigenous cultures who value natural remedies. Sometimes you might be surprised as to who those folks are. My (Adenike's) mother was a physician. At one point she had a private practice, she worked for the ministry of health in Trinidad, and helmed various public health initiatives when she worked with the Pan American Health Organization. She often read medical journals, and she belonged to medical societies and associations where she could learn about and discuss developing research and treatments. With all of that scientific knowledge, her go-to treatment was gargling with warm salt water. No matter if my cough was just a tickle due to dry air or if my sneeze was because of dust, if Mummy heard anything she could deem a symptom of possible ill health, she'd ask, "Did you gargle with warm salt water?"

As much as I teased my mother about her remedy, if I take a good look at my family's approach to promoting well-being, natural remedies have played a huge part in it. My grandmother believed that baking soda was the best thing on G-d's green earth. She used it for insect bites, deodorant, and toothpaste if we ran out. And I'm no different when it comes to tea. The moment I feel any sort of stomachache or anyone around me says they feel poorly, I run to the cabinet to pull out ginger tea, mint tea or, if we're really lucky or it's a serious situation, ginger-mint tea.

In many parts of the Caribbean, "bush" tea is a huge part of curing various symptoms ranging from upset stomach and fevers to aches and pains.[10] I grew up in Trinidad hearing about people in my family and community who drank orange peel tea, fever grass tea, or caraille tea. Add to that some "soft candle" to rub on painful joints or aching muscles and you're good to go! Regardless of my community's ability to afford pharmacological drugs, using the natural remedies available in our backyards and that were passed down to us by our Ancestors was an important way of affirming our cultural identity and our cultural understandings of health and well-being.

The thing about western/European medicine isn't that it doesn't save lives or that it doesn't improve the quality of life for people regardless of their cultural origins. Remember, every thread in our human tapestry holds value! The thing that causes damage is holding up and relying too heavily on one single thread to be the only or best way of promoting and maintaining health. This is the thing that is one-sided, and even dangerous, in some situations. For a large number of people across the Diaspora, the western/European worldview invalidates their lived experience of healing and well-being, and can be deadly.[11] Reclaiming African healing traditions that embody a wholistic understanding of personhood is one way to more sustainably move towards liberation. The remedies and practices that our Ancestors relied on for centuries still have value, and lifting them up alongside more recently woven threads supports the overall strength of the tapestry. Learning about Ancestral practices and engaging with them in a manner that is relevant for our current contexts will help us re-member ourselves, our histories, and our identity.

Tap in for Reflection: Connect the Threads between Our Ancestral and Bodily Knowings

It's time to begin getting really clear about the throughlines we've identified thus far. We're going to take this time to look back at the first two sections of this book and identify some spaces/resources we will need to consult for the final section to come.

1. Go back to your answers from the exercise "Tap in for Reflection: Build Your Own Ancestral Wisdoms List," in Section 1, Chapter 4. Make note of any Ancestral Wisdoms relating to natural remedies (foods, herbs, etc.) or other healing practices (praying, grief rituals, etc.).
    a. You may wish to do this on an all-new sheet of paper, so you don't have to keep flipping back and forth between this and the information you're about to locate next.

2. Now find the exercise "Pour into Practice: Breathe into Your Connection(s)" from Section 2, Chapter 5. Revisit the Connection Gesture you arrived at for representing your connection to the Motherland.
    a. If you were someone who chose to put on a piece of music and dance, record yourself doing it again, then view the video and write down brief/basic descriptions of any moments that stand out to you. Or if you showed this movement to someone else, go back to that person and ask them to describe what they remember of the movement and/or conversation about it, and write down whatever stands out to you from that moment of recollection.
    b. Ideally, you'll write these descriptions down on the same piece of paper as the one you just wrote your revisited Ancestral Wisdoms on.

3. Ask yourself: What lives between what I've written about

my Ancestral Wisdoms and what I've written about my connection to Africa?

a. You may identify feelings you have/had that are similar in both exercises, or common words/themes you used in your responses, or you may see no connection whatsoever. Either way, this is data you can use!
   i. If you identify common feelings, words, or themes, find a way to identify and/or tie them together, either by highlighting them all in the same color or literally drawing a line between them.
   ii. If you see no connection whatsoever, write this down: "I do not yet see a thread between my Ancestral Wisdoms and what I have written of my connection to Africa." That word—"yet"—is important, because we aim to remedy the situation around it!

Here we pause to share an example that may be helpful. My (Natasha's) father used to make a Caribbean treat we just called "sugarcake." I reference this treat in a book chapter I co-wrote with Nsamu Moonga for the second edition of the *Handbook of Music Therapy* as a familial comfort food which I would definitely include on a list of Ancestral Wisdoms (because comfort foods can absolutely be medicine!).[12] In that chapter, I speak about feelings I experienced in 2021 on finding the exact recipe for that sugarcake in a Yoruban cookbook, listed as a dish frequently served in offering to the Orisha (spirit) Yemoja, sometimes referred to as "Mother of All." I describe it similarly to the "ecstatic grief" I referred to in the opening of this book. But what I didn't say in that book was that a small representation of Yemoya has sat on the mantle of every house I've lived in since 2013, almost a decade prior, when my journey of integrating more Afro-Diasporic practices into my life began. Never in that time did I believe my family or Ancestors to have any specific historical connection to that Orisha. I just felt in my bones somehow that out of the many I've learned about over the years, Yemoya has held special meaning to me, even if I couldn't understand why in the beginning. Knowing what I know now, it's like my family's recipe has held this "secret" link to Yemoya for multiple generations. If I were to put that feeling of connection into a gesture, similar to the Chapter 5 exercise "Pour into Practice: Breathe into Your Connection(s)," it would be a gesture similar to the one that a person's arms make when they are treading water, a sort of cyclical motion with both arms at chest level, moving the water around me, while the rest of my body stays still. If I were to put this into writing in the way I've encouraged you to do above, it might look like this:

Ancestral Practice	My Connection Gesture	Ancestral Wisdom
The making of sugarcake—a familial comfort food	Treading water—a way to stay alive	Comfort food can be medicine—medicine can be a way to stay alive. This is the thread between my Ancestral Wisdom and my Connection Gesture. This is what connects me to Africa. My Ancestral Body knows many ways to stay alive.

Now let's take this a little deeper.

Pour into Practice: Prepare to Act on your Connections!

1. Whether you identified a connection in the above reflection exercise or not, you're going to write a declarative sentence about what your Ancestral Body knows.
    a. My example above merges my Ancestral Wisdom with my Connection Gesture, reading: "My Ancestral Body knows many ways to stay alive." Yours might do the same, or...
    b. ...if you couldn't identify a connection, or the connection you identified doesn't easily fit into the sentence structure we've invited above, you can craft your defining statement from either the Ancestral Wisdom or the

Connection Gesture that you identified, because both of those things are knowledges held by your body today!

2. You are going to craft this knowledge statement into a task—a sort of "next step" to undertake. To help you get there, you're going to use the following formulaic sentence: "I want to learn more about the ways my Ancestors . . . ."
   a. As an example, my task might read: "I want to learn more about the ways my Ancestors stayed alive."
   b. Read your task back to yourself and feel how your body reacts. For me, I feel my head sort of cocking to one side like, "That doesn't read quite the way I want it to." You can follow those kinds of signals! With a little tweaking, I've revised my task to: "I want to learn more about the ways my Ancestors sustained themselves."

It is important to note here that the task you assign for yourself may lead you into more complicated places, like wanting to know more about your Ancestors' responsibility for certain atrocities, or you may find yourself articulating a task that leads you to somewhere further away from Africa; all of that is ok in this moment! Whether or not your thread brings you closer to the continent in the ways you want or expect, you have just articulated a path towards strengthening a thread of connection that you either didn't have before or couldn't clearly articulate until this moment invited you to do so. You are already on your way to making the tapestry of your lineage stronger. So remember, if something has not been uncovered or healed (yet!), it doesn't mean it can't be uncovered or healed later! All things in their time.

Onward.

Chapter 7

What We Hold in Our Bodies

When we consider all the impacts of western/colonial policies of exploitation, dehumanization, and subjugation on our bodies, minds and spirits, we find ourselves at a critical intersection: a place of pause and acknowledgement. We want to sit in that place just a little while longer here, with deep intentionality, in order to identify our most effective and sustainable path forward.

Tap in for Reflection: Sit with the Complexity of Your Ancestral Body's Task

1. Find a place and time where you can sit comfortably. Take a moment to get tuned in to your environment and your breath, without judgment. Just notice the sights, sounds, and cadences of your body in this moment.

2. Close your eyes and do a brief scan of your body, similar to the "Somatic Self-Portraits" exercise in "Pour into Practice: Attune to Your Sense of Bodily Knowing" but without the writing/drawing tools, just making note of any tension or other state of being in your body that feels important to track.

3. Find and reread the task you identified for yourself in "Pour

into Practice: Prepare to Act on your Connections!" As you read it, pay attention to your body, and anything that may shift or respond to reviewing your task.

   a. For reference, the one I (Natasha) had identified for myself was: "I want to learn more about the ways my Ancestors sustained themselves."
   b. Make note of anything that shifts or changes.

4. You're going to turn any noted shifts or changes into subtasks for yourself. Take a moment to reformulate them as such by adding a phrase like: "I want to know more about this shift that happens when I think about my task."
   a. If you didn't note any shifts, that's still data you can track! You can note: "I want to know more about the lack of shifts I feel when I think about my task."

5. Also consider any prerequisite or clarifying actions that your task may require. For instance, in order for me to know more about the way my Ancestors sustained themselves, I need to know who my Ancestors were and what part(s) of the world they were situated in. Finding out who my Ancestors were may require speaking to specific people or looking up/subscribing to a service to help me on my way. Each of those needs is a new task, yielding new information that will then require processing into additional tasks, like identifying a specific group of Ancestors to focus my attention on rather than trying to take them all on at once.
   a. As you note each of these prerequisites or clarifying actions, do additional scans to catch any extra shifts or changes that may be needed to add to your (hopefully) growing list of subtasks.

What we're doing here is allowing your initial task to be complicated. To live in more than one place. All too often we assign ourselves tasks that become solely intellectual exercises. "I want to know more about something" takes us into books and conversations that may be valuable, but we also want to be consulting our own bodies as resources as well!

Here is another layer of complexity to consider as well: everything we are encouraging you to do here is going to need to be tested in multiple contexts. What you learn in your body will need to be weighed against the historical information you may find and then re-integrated into your body. After that re-integration you'll need to measure it again within your current environment, re-integrate once more, and then venture into measuring it anew within your current relationships. Breathe. This will not be a fast or linear thing. It may not be an easy thing either. We are, after all, asking you to consider a task that is situated within your entire Ancestral lineage and all the complex human history surrounding it! Breathe. One step at a time.

Parallels between Indigenous Peoples and Wisdoms across Time and Space

When I (Natasha) sit with the complexity of taking on a task such as learning more about my Ancestors' way of sustaining themselves, some of the tasks I've uncovered and undertaken for myself have included:

- revisiting my old Ancestry.com DNA testing results from 2014:
  - subtask: researching how to remove my data from that site once I'm done with it so they can't sell it!
  - subtask: deciding which branch of my DNA testing to follow up on (I chose to narrow my focus on Africa first and then revisit my European results later)
  - subtask: learning more about the shifts I feel when I think about my African results vs. my European results

- signing up for AfricanAncestry.com to get additional DNA testing that can tell me more about the tribal groups my people came from (and celebrating the fact that that service destroys my data for me after I've received my results)

- joining an online community of people relevant to the tribal groups identified for me by my DNA results, which includes:
  - finding and communicating with people like me, looking to get re-connected, in person where possible
    - > subtask: sitting with the shifts in my body that arise with each interaction I've had thus far
  - getting to know the people and practices living within those tribal groups today (this is the step I'm currently in the middle of).

Some of what I've learned so far has been that the people living in the tribal groups that I am descended from today share a great many parallel experiences to the Indigenous peoples of Turtle Island, where I am currently situated, as well as my own existing Ancestral Body's knowings. This has yielded a lot of complexity for me, particularly around my Queerness and the impact of colonization on the way people who identify under the LGBTQIA+ umbrella are perceived and engaged with. Similar to western perspectives on health, colonizing beliefs about sex and gender hold a great many "rules" that are ultimately grounded in the idea of certainty (i.e., "If I see a person with XYZ body parts then this-thing-I've-internalized-about-gender-roles *must* be the place they hold in society and there are *never* exceptions to this because this thing I learned has been passed down as knowledge that can never be questioned!"). The impact of this colonial framing can be seen in anti-Queer beliefs and practices being upheld by some living Indigenous peoples, as well as those seeking to re-integrate with their Ancestral lineages. This can be as subtle as coded cultural messaging that promotes non-disclosure (aka "closeting," which is just another way to say "hiding") of any "behavior" which may be considered "controversial" (which usually means Queer). For instance, I have found in some groups I've connected with that I can bring a same-sex partner to a tribal gathering if I want to (yay!), but I shouldn't introduce them as such, lest it "upset" anyone present (no thank you!). Then there are outright laws against homosexuality in some African countries that may result in someone being imprisoned, tortured, or killed if they are reported. These are beliefs and practices that have been promoted and bolstered by western/colonial interference and insidiously fed to the Indigenous peoples of the land. We want to be clear in stating here that hatred and derision of Queerness is not historically or culturally accurate to our peoples' Ancestral ways!

There are multiple notable instances of historical Queerness across the African Diaspora.[1] [2] What I (Natasha) have found in my own exploration and learning is that they were just never labeled as such because our Ancestors didn't need to label them. Herein lie the nuance and complexity, and Queerness is just one among many examples of how complex our histories are.[3] As one example, I found in my studies a piece of work about "lesbianism" in the Themne peoples who were enslaved in the Caribbean, as my Ancestors were. The labeling of this "homosexual behavior" was placed by researchers long after the fact as a description of something that was common practice on the African continent, and it only became a covert (hidden) practice in the wake of slavery when it became critical for people assigned female at birth to protect each other whenever their husbands were away (whether sold away from the family during enslavement or after slavery, when many men were forced to work jobs at sea that might have them away for months at a time). These women would form what some folks today would call "pods" by planning to marry into the same family (each marrying a brother or a cousin, for example), so no one would question them moving in together when their husbands were out of the picture. Many times, the husbands were totally aware this was happening, and had no problems with it, such that it didn't need to be defined or labeled the way we do now. What is complicated about this is that we (the Black/African Diasporic descendants of today) live in a world where this kind of history is constantly being hidden or erased, and so naming ourselves, our practices, and our ways of being, and sharing them loudly, is for many an important act of rebellion against systems of harm.

This naming has come at great cost.[4] Colonizers have historically gone to significant and horrific lengths to punish Queer "behavior," often enacting that punishment on any/all people who knew about it as well, in order to discourage its continuance in any form, even discussion. This is part of how genocide works: if you wish to fully kill a people, you have to kill not only their bodies but their histories too.

There are, of course, more layers to this that Black Queer folks will know or sense between the lines of this book (because remember, we sometimes just know stuff without saying it!). We know that part of the effort to kill Indigenous histories has also involved encouraging people to police any form of "other"ness within our own ranks by turning on each other, believing it will protect the majority. And it is also true that western/colonial practices have been so insidious in so many ways that it is understandable why some peoples would question language or ways of being in the world that they perceive to be "new" if they've had parts of their history erased or hidden from them. So untangling a lot of our peoples' perspectives on Queerness is incredibly complex, and not something anyone should expect or set out to do alone, let alone quickly or easily!

See why sitting with complexity is important? The work of colonization took generations to enact. It will take generations to undo. Breathe, and do what you can with the body/mind/capacity you have right now, in this moment.

For me (Natasha) right now, I am continuing to sit with how anti-Queer language and practices among my peoples, knowing that this wasn't always our way, brings me fresh grief each time I experience it. This has taken time for me to fully feel into. And, as time has passed, I am finding my way through my feelings towards the people and spaces I need to connect further with. Queer folks in many parts of the world today use a combination of coded and overt language to help us articulate what we know about ourselves and find each other in critical ways that keep us safe. Learning about these people, spaces, and practices can sometimes feel like learning a new language. Community organizers and historians Stephen Murray, Will Roscoe, and others like those behind the YouTube channel "Documenting Queerness," which includes interviews with elders in countries like Ghana, are doing incredible work documenting the words and lives of Queer folks throughout history, in order to ensure there is a record of the way African Queerness has existed throughout history, including pre-colonization.[5] These are the kind of people I am working to get more connected to so that I can continue my efforts at getting re-integrated into my peoples, with respect for their current context, while also staying true to myself and who I know myself to be: someone my Ancestors would (and do!) love, just as I am.

The Delicate Nature of Space and Re-Traumatization

As we talk about what our bodies have held historically, and what we know of them now, it's important to recognize what they hold right now as we think about ongoing, pervasive harm at community and family levels. As I (Adenike) write these words, I feel almost short of breath and anxious. I feel my shoulders rising and tension in my arms and chest. I want to curl in on myself and run away, removing myself from the weight of centuries of harm that my family and my community have carried. If you are feeling anything similar, I invite you to pause and check in with your body.

Tap in for Reflection: (Re)Ground in Your Physical Senses and Environment

Feel your feet planted on the floor or supported by what you're sitting or resting on. Touch what's beside you, like a table, pillow, or the floor. Inhale slowly and deeply. Exhale slowly and completely. Notice three objects in the room you're in, and name them out loud.

For me, I see a small, green ceramic plant pot, an old toy stuffed dog, and my red-handled pair of scissors. Inhale slowly and deeply. Exhale slowly and completely. Look around you, above you, and behind you. Reassure yourself that you are safe. Inhale slowly and deeply. Exhale slowly and completely.

When we realize that we've been carrying trauma in our family heritage or our cultural group, it can bring up a range of emotions. Some of those we might feel ready to acknowledge and express. Some of those we might want to avoid or push down even more. We might want to spring into action mode and get to the root of the trauma and yank it out of our lives. All that is normal; however, it's important to remember a couple of things:

- Avoiding difficult or painful emotions takes a toll on us after a while in ways that we may not anticipate. It's ok if you don't have the capacity to fully explore or deal with something right now, but make sure you have a way to do that sooner rather than later. Maybe your reactions to reading this motivate you to seek professional counseling or therapy, or to connect with a spiritual advisor or trusted friend. Identify what could help you when you're ready to dive deeper.

- Intergenerational trauma develops over centuries, so it's highly unlikely that you will be able to uproot it from your life overnight or even in a few months. Give yourself time to acknowledge what you feel and think as you continue to learn more about your family or culture's experiences. Give yourself time to identify supports and resources to help you heal. And give yourself time to heal.

An important part of healing intergenerational trauma involves recognizing your role in the healing process. You cannot undo what one of your Ancestors did 5 or 20 generations ago. You cannot undo what your community did 200 years ago. You are responsible for what happens now, informed by those histories, and going forward. To figure that out, you'll need to ask yourself some serious questions.

Tap in for Reflection: Begin to Strategize about Your Familial/Community Environment (and Possible Collaborators on Your Healing Journey!)

Take some time to journal on the following prompts:

- How do you generally engage as a member of your family and/or community with other family/community members?

  - Is this how you want/choose to engage? If so, describe some elements of what you do that you want to ensure you keep doing. If not, that's ok, just sit with that awareness.

- What are some patterns that you see repeating over and over again in your family/community, whether they are patterns of behavior or things that seem to follow or keep happening? Pay particular attention to any patterns that may cause difficulty for your family/community, pausing to reground in your physical environment, and be gentle with yourself as needed!
  - Identify what elements of those patterns you can control. What might be necessary for you to do or change so that you don't perpetuate patterns of harm within your family/community?

- Who can you share this with in your family/community at this time, in order to invite them to walk beside you in a collaborative healing journey?
  - If you can't identify anyone who would be safe for you to do this with at this time, who might be safe for you to do this with in the future, if you were able to build a little more trust? Or is this something that you might need to reach outside your immediate family/community to connect with someone over?

- How else might you learn what is needed for your family/community to recover from harm?

- Is there anyone else (whether a person or an organization) you can partner with?

What is being invited here is a precursor to pod-mapping, as first described by Bay Area Transformative Justice.[6] In pod-mapping, we use networks of connected circles to identify people and agencies close to us to whom we might turn in times of crisis or need. Different gradients of lines or colors can be used to identify people or orgs (organizations) you feel closest to, as distinguished from those who you might need more trust or time to feel closer to or safer with. If you wish, you can use the sample map below to turn your journaling above into a more graphic pod-map.

Pour into Practice: Convert Your Journaling into a Pod-Map!

A template crafted by Natasha sits below this text. In the center of the image, a circle with a little curl above it is meant to hold your name, with solid spirals surrounding it. Those are intended for the names of those people or orgs closest to you in trusting relationship. These may or may not be people or orgs that live or operate physically close to you, but you may wish to make different maps to distinguish your "neighborhood" pod from other collections of people/orgs.

Encircling all the solid spirals are circles framed with dashed lines. Those indicate people or orgs with whom you may need more trust or time to feel more firmly connected. Along the edges of the image are curved lines, dashes, and squiggles forming a border. The different textures in those lines/dashes/squiggles are not just aesthetic in nature but can also be used as suggestions for lines you can draw between circles to indicate the different ways each one may be connected to you (blood relatives, neighbors, friends, etc.). Of course, you can also create your own textures and keys for this map as well!

A larger version of this image can be found in the accompanying workbook.

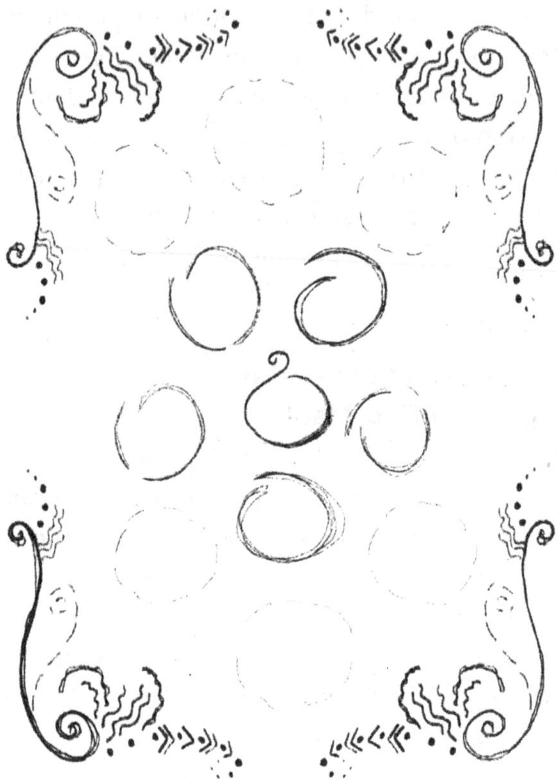

Remember, as you note these people and agencies to which you are (or could be) connected, you can only do what it is your healing work to do. You can't force someone to understand or change something if they are not ready to do that or receptive to even admitting that it needs to happen. You are not responsible for healing or saving others. Sometimes focusing on "helping" others is a way we make ourselves feel better and less accountable for the harm we've contributed to. But remember, that is not what is needed here. What is needed is being real about where we are now, recognizing how it connects to the past, and then bridging those connections towards the mutual benefit and liberation of all those we are connected to. Whether those on the other sides of the bridges we build actually manage to walk all the way across them is not something we should expect or force.

Focus instead on finding your place in the sea of humanity that is always moving, growing, and learning, and move alongside those you find near you on your journey. As you may have noted in your risks and rewards in "Pour into Practice: Calculate Your 'Risks and Rewards'" in Section 1, this may mean that you lose some people or get left behind by others. Breathe through it all, and open yourself to the possibilities that you will gain more than you lose.

Whether you are aware of all the people moving in the same direction as you from moment to moment, know that there are oh so many of us! We walk shoulder to shoulder, forward, and across many planes, together.

Section Review

In this section, we have discussed current realities of colonization and possible Black-affirming avenues for healing and creativity within those realities, including:

- deepening our understanding of why centering Black folks in liberation work is important
- specific ways western medicine stifles cultural and bodily knowledge
- the importance of contextualizing ourselves and our work in Ancestrally affirming ways.

We have undertaken an increasing number of reflections and practices in order to build on the work we began in Section 1:

1. Reflect: Define Your Connection to Africa
   a. Practice: Breathe into Your Connection(s)

2. Reflect: Contextualize Your Experience of Pain
   a. Practice: Poetic (Re)Construction

3. Reflect: Stories of the Inexplicable in Health
   a. Practice: Attune to Your Sense of Bodily Knowing

4. Reflect: Connect the Threads between Our Ancestral and Bodily Knowings
    a. Practice: Prepare to Act on your Connections!

5. Reflect: Sit with the Complexity of Your Ancestral Body's Task

6. Reflect: (Re)Ground in Your Physical Senses and Environment

7. Reflect: Begin to Strategize about Your Familial/Community Environment (and Possible Collaborators on Your Healing Journey!)
    a. Practice: Convert Your Journaling into a Pod-Map!

Below is a possible schedule for integrating these practices into your life on a regular basis, infusing them alongside/between the practices recommended in Section 1:

<table>
<tr><th>Daily</th><th>Weekly</th><th>Monthly</th><th>As you feel led</th></tr>
<tr><td>Describe sensations (from Section 1)</td><td>Tend an Ancestral space (from Section 1)</td><td>(Re)calculate risks and rewards (from Section 1)</td><td>Re(define) your connection to Africa, breathe into what's newly emerging or able to be released</td></tr>
<tr><td colspan="2">(Re)ground in your physical environment

Check in on your Ancestral/bodily connections and tasks: How would you define where you are in your journey right now? What progress are you making? What feels important to make note of or adjust?</td><td>(Re)contextualize your experience of pain (or another sensation you can identify and feel led to explore!)</td><td>Poetic (re) construction of any previous exercise: When you look back at what you've constructed, what do you feel led to play with or explore more deeply?</td></tr>
<tr><td>Tune into Dreamspace (from section 1)</td><td></td><td>Revisit your familial/ community context journaling and/or pod-map!</td><td></td></tr>
</table>

Section 3

DREAMING INTO WHAT IS POSSIBLE

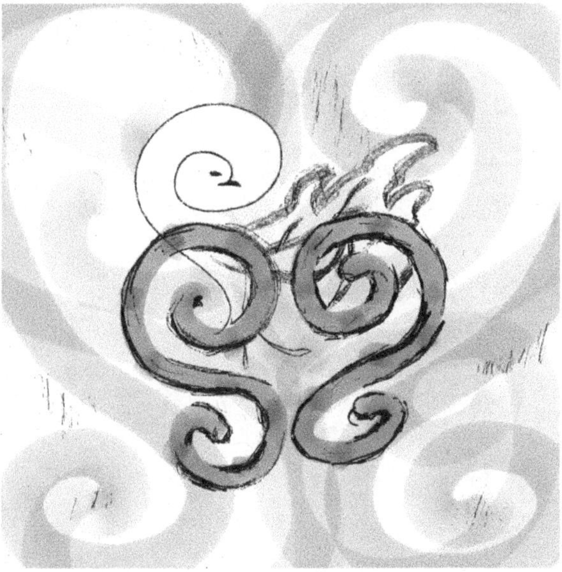

Chapter 8

Weaving Together Past/Present/Future, and Body/Mind/Spirit

In the waking hours of 2023, I (Natasha) had a dream that would eventually lead to the creation of BCH's regular internal (Black-only) meeting schedule, including a free monthly social hour, a creative co-working session (also free of charge), and the establishment of a multiracial Patreon space, which folks from any racial background could subscribe to for as little as $5 a month. My dream also—unbeknownst to me at the time—was the initial catalyst for the Black Creative Healing Album, which we released as an EP in late 2024. As of this writing, more music is planned for late 2026/early 2027.

Having already established a practice of documenting my dreams (as we've encouraged you to do in Section 1 of this book!), I inscribed the entirety of the dream and followed up on the experience by crafting visual images to accompany the story of it, eventually sharing the story and images with subscribers to the BCH Patreon in the summer of 2023. An abbreviated version of the dream's story would eventually make it into the early 2025 music video for the first track of the BCH EP, titled "Prelude (Join Us)." I encourage listening to that track, and the EP as a whole, during this section of the book if you feel so led!

In the dream, I was encouraged by a dark-skinned African priest to step into a pool of water and follow its current down a path to a door. When I opened the door, I found myself in a room full of tools, which I didn't describe in the music video but elaborated on more for our Patreon, as well as for folks in our Black-only Discord/Zoom spaces. The specific nature of the tools isn't particularly important. What's important is that seeing those tools held meaning for me; I had associations with the purpose they served. That purpose encouraged me to begin thinking about how (and what!) I was serving my community. It led me to begin more mindfully encouraging regular gatherings and opportunities for collective creative energies to be stirred into being.

We initially promoted our social hours and a few workshop-style events via Eventbrite, where people could register for free and then fill out a survey to confirm their registration. The survey proved to be critical to the success of our gatherings, as it helped us rule out bots and people who hadn't really given any thought to why they might want to join a healing space, or for whom our space might not otherwise be right for their needs. Adenike and I would review each survey response, and then reply to each individual who filled it out, sharing with them the links to the appropriate space for them (whether Discord or Patreon) and the Zoom link to the relevant gathering when we felt comfortable doing so. By the end of 2023, we had a group of people who were showing up with increasing regularity to our events, and we made the choice late in that year to close down the public invitation space on Eventbrite in order to focus on deepening our relationships with more intentionality. The Patreon space continues to be active; we just don't promote it the same way we used to. Our Black-only spaces are prioritized first, with automated reminders for our events going out regularly to those community members and additional events/offerings being made in our Patreon and/or more public spaces (website, social media, etc.) as Adenike's and my capacity allows.

During the Black-only social hours of 2023, we got to know each other: where we lived, what we did for our creative practices, what impact creativity had on our lives, etc. Then during the creative co-works, we would log into Zoom and set intentions for our time together, including what each of us wanted to work on in our own spaces, and then we would turn our cameras off, mute ourselves, and simply work alongside each other in the virtual sphere, each of us creating in our own ways/times for roughly an hour, and then returning to conversation, where we would share what we'd made and any lessons or feelings that were sitting with us about what we'd done or created.

Our gatherings very quickly took on a sort of sacredness. As one participant put it, we didn't always know what we were getting when we logged in to meet, but we always knew it would be something beautiful, and something we needed. As of this writing in late 2024/early 2025, our Discord and Zoom spaces are by invitation only, and I'm not sure when or if that will ever change. It feels important for that community to grow with care, or not at all. But grow it has! Every once in a while, Adenike or I will meet someone at an event or in our community who feels kindred to us, and after a brief period of consulting with each other, we send out links of invitation as we feel so led, and the process of getting to know each other more deeply continues.

Our Patreon can be joined by anyone (Black or non-Black) at any time and serves as our main public interactive space (aside from our social media spaces and occasional presentations or events that Adenike and/or I do in collaboration with other orgs). Adenike and I share journaling reflections or art in progress and occasionally conduct events where folks from our Patreon and Discord spaces can interact with each other via Zoom. In time, we may do more public events or series that are even more interactive, but for now, our current gradient of spaces offers our community multitiered points of access for grounding ourselves in creativity, exploring concepts of solidarity with each other, and engaging in critical reflection on our everyday practices and beliefs. This is the kind of deep healing work that we believe contributes to the more liberated world we want to see.

The Role of Ritual

Similar to discussion of altars, bringing up the concept of ritual can raise some hackles for folks. Our western conditioning would have us believe that rituals are big, intense, and intimidating things that are only ever attached to a religious practice or context, otherwise they are either irrelevant to our lives or best to be avoided. Of course, as we've been sharing in this book, our Ancestral and Indigenous Wisdoms know otherwise! Anything we find ourselves turning to with deep intention and/or doing again and again is a ritual: a family reunion can be a ritual, work can be ritual, waking and bedtime routines can be rituals. All that is needed to give strength to a ritual is the intentionality with which we approach it.

Both Ancestor Malidoma Patrice Some and his wife, Sobonfu Some, present beautiful portraits of ritual work in descriptions of everyday life growing up among the Dagara peoples of Burkina Faso, translating it for western audiences.[1] As an example, Malidoma speaks of his mother singing as she milled grain for up to six hours a day, a practice that helped her to pass the time but also served as a sort of intention-building in her work. He describes the meals made with the milled grain as being that much more nourishing because of the devotion the whole family knew had been poured into the work.

Tap in for Reflection: Acknowledge Your Rituals, (Re)Assess Associations with Spirituality

What are some rituals that you engage in regularly for yourself? You can list anything, from the mundane/everyday, like brushing your teeth, to maybe some newer practices you have taken on from this book. You don't need to list every ritual you can think of, just a few that feel important to name.

Once you have populated a small list, revisit the reflection you made on spirituality in Chapter 4 in "Tap in for Reflection: Assess Your Associations with Spirituality." Note anything that has changed (or may be shifting/deepening) in your associations with spiritual practice.

Returning to reflection on the regular gatherings that BCH has in its Black-only spaces, and even the broader Patreon or public event spaces we curate, the intentionality of ritual is very present. We begin with gentle grounding, often asking some sort of predetermined check-in question or (if it is a larger group) inviting folks to get situated in their bodies before we begin. Some of the ways we invite this situating in the body may include:

- placing your feet flat on the floor, or at least becoming aware of how your body is situated against surfaces it may be touching

- becoming aware of your breath

- doing an internal scan of your body for any places you may be feeling tension, fatigue, or other sensations:
  - meeting any needs that may arise in your body by bringing warmth to them with your hands or adjusting your positioning
  - we may also encourage taking a moment to grab water, tea, or a snack to have nearby in case folks feel a need to nourish their bodies in those ways as we progress.

Many of these are invitations you may have seen us make in this book! They are practices that feel almost second nature to me (Natasha) now, but something else I have noted is that if I am in a meeting where these actions are not explicitly encouraged, my body/mind will still forget them and revert to old conditioning that says, "Don't you move a muscle—give this room all your attention!" So I have come to think of the naming of the body, and encouragement to meet its needs, as part of the ritual, and it is something I sometimes have to do silently for myself if I am in a space that doesn't seem open to pausing for it. I share this here as a moment of reflecting my own process in progress, a reminder that none of us is perfect, and an invitation and encouragement to find the ways that work most authentically for you to remind yourself to return to your body whenever you can—it's never too late to check back in!

Something that also feels valuable to name here is how ritual often mirrors creative process as well. We may enter with our box of tools and predetermined intentions, but there is always a point where, as Malidoma describes it, "the (ritual) journey owns you,"[2] and you are moving through the work on instinct or feeling alone. This is also described by Mihaly Csikszentmihalyi,[3] who studies the concept of happiness, as a state of "flow:" it is a place most accessible when someone who possesses a great deal of experience in something meets the place where spontaneity can take over. It takes practice to find flow! That is part of what this book has been encouraging you to find as well, particularly as we progress further into this idea of building on the more liberated world we are imagining.

Pour into Practice: Making Time for "Flow"

Take a moment to look back at the Pouring into Practice exercises from Sections 1 and 2 (yes, all of them!). We have gradually been encouraging deeper and more extended creative action, from small gestures/doodles, writing exercises, and playlist-building, to larger scale drawing, movement, and poetic (re)construction.

As you review those invitations and your responses to them, is there a particular practice that you can identify where you most felt your body in a state of flow? That is to say, a place where your body felt confident enough in its ability to do what was being asked of you such that the result seemed to pour from you with seemingly minimal effort, or where you may have been so invested in the process that you lost track of the time? Make note of those practices and categorize them in your mind, or on paper, using terms that feel most authentic to you.

As an example, Natasha most easily enters flow state when singing, but small-scale movement is also a place where it can happen. So "singing" and "small-scale movement" would be her terms.

Once you've identified those practices, take a look at your schedule for the next week. Where might you make time to dive into a flow sometime in the next seven days? You may have to do some planning here, like thinking about how much time you'll need, where might be the best place to dive in, and what tools you may need to have with you. We will bring you into the practice itself in a later exercise, but just for today, make a plan.

Lastly, identify someone who you can consider your

accountability buddy for this plan. Maybe it's a family member or friend you plan to do the work with, or speak to afterwards about it, or maybe you locate a craft circle or other creative co-work type of environment, where the other people in attendance might serve as the people who can affirm your presence/commitment to the work. Make sure that some aspect of your community is part of your plan!

Something you may be noticing is that the invitations we are making for your reflection and practice are a little more sparse than in previous sections. This is in part because we assume that if practices from earlier sections have been slowly getting integrated into your life, you may be glad of not having too much more complexity to be marinating at the same time. But also, these invitations are more sparse because this is the place where we are beginning to take the training wheels off a little bit and want to empower your deepening sense of self-knowing to start taking over, such that you don't need as much detail or prompting from us to enter creative practice. You are becoming the expert in your own healing journey!

Chapter 9

Reflexivity, Solidarity, and Staying Grounded

Our African Ancestors lived in a state of mutuality and reciprocity. In many cultures across the continent, communities and relationships were structured around the principle/concept of what several Bantu-speaking cultures refer to as *ubuntu*—"I am because we are." Our humanity exists in the context of being connected to greater physical, environmental, and spiritual communities. Cutting ourselves off from each other, from these communities, cuts us off from what makes us really human. This isn't to say that our Ancestors always maintained perfectly harmonious relationships in every aspect of their lives. Wars happened. Betrayals happened. Slavery happened. Yet our Ancestors were continually called back to living in the way of *ubuntu*, as that was how their communities were designed. Living this way reminds members of the community that they are no greater or lesser than anyone else. That, "I exist and have value because you exist." That, "I thrive because you thrive." My freedom and ability to live into my full potential is interwoven with your freedom and your ability to live into your full potential. This is the grounding for liberation, and for healing, that we must return to and tend, again and again.

The entry points from which we return may not be the same every time, like entering a spiral staircase from a different floor. But each new entrance should yield valuable perspectives and possibilities that can be made even stronger when we can take the time to continually map and assess how each new thing we learn or experience relates to, or differs from, the one before.

My (Adenike's) journey to BCH began with Oprah. When I finished my PhD, my sister gave me a copy of Oprah's book, *The Path Made Clear*, a collection of reflections about discovering your purpose and inspirational quotes by renowned leaders. I decided to read a chapter every day and write any reflections in my journal. During my journaling one day, I took a moment to imagine how my life's purpose could be expressed. The idea of having a podcast popped into my head. At that stage in my life, I had yet to ever listen to one! I sort of chuckled at my flight of fantasy and went about my day. About eight months later, Natasha shared that she was looking to pivot her conversations with Black Creatives from a video format to a podcast and that she'd like to have someone co-host it with her. Without a second of hesitation (and with no clue what that would entail!), I said I'd do it. As a result, over the past four years, I have developed a more expansive and meaningful understanding of what it is for me to be well. My journey of integrative healing would be incomplete without those conversations with Black Creatives, sharing arts-based reflections, and making space regularly for Black-identifying members of the African Diaspora to meet and create together. My experience as part of BCH has opened my eyes to the power of being reflexive, creating community, and continually re-connecting with my embodied values and wisdom.

Some people say that there are no coincidences or accidents; I'm inclined to agree with them. The BCH podcast began during the first year of the COVID-19 pandemic. The "two-week" lockdown that began in March 2020 was still going strong when we produced our first episode in June. So many of us were experiencing feelings of isolation, being disconnected, depression, and other aspects of diminished well-being. Several surveys and many anecdotes about the impact of lockdown pointed out that in the United States, Black people experienced greater hardship compared with other groups.[1 2] The fact that our podcast, which focuses on how members of Black communities promote and sustain healing and well-being, came to life at that particular time feels significant to me. So much happened in 2020. In addition to the existential threat of the pandemic, there was the great civil unrest in response to the murder of George

Floyd by Minneapolis police. Black bodies were under siege in more ways than one. Black spirits were being diminished in more ways than one. Our focus on healing through collaborative creative processes became a necessary response, an important way to remind each other that we weren't as disconnected, worthless, or powerless as various oppressive systems would have us be. Connecting with Black Creatives doing the work of supporting well-being and fighting injustice was a form of solidarity. Sharing ideas on how to explore facets of our social lives, psychological lives, and spiritual lives by engaging in our creativity was one way to support collective efforts of Black liberation.

Doing this work has not been without its challenges. All work requires energy to complete, and when you're not being paid for your labor, that can make it harder to find time for. Both of us have been privileged enough that at various points in our career, our academic day jobs paid for the time we poured into BCH as part of our research agendas and community service. We have also been fortunate enough to receive a few grants and donations (like the ones through our Patreon) that have helped support our ability to pay facilitators (including ourselves) for events over time, like the BCH retreat, which would not have been possible without the support of the Black Music Therapy Network, catalyzed by our dear friend Marisol Norris. Now, while I (Natasha) no longer teach full time, or have a day job that pays for my time to pour into BCH the way I used to, I am tremendously grateful that our small-but-mighty Patreon following allows us to at least sustain our monthly internal events, and I am continuously humbled and elated at opportunities that have arisen from relationships we've developed over time with other people, projects, and orgs who have been able to host us as paid facilitators for their events.

This is the ground floor of reflexivity and solidarity. We take the time, over and over, to reflect on how we got where we are and who helped us get here. As we build new relationships, we honor the ones that preceded them, and always hold their needs close to us, extending care as we make decisions about how we want to move next.

Pour into Practice: Take a Moment to Say Thank You!
Who can you reach out to today to say thank you for their impact on your healing journey? Take a moment to make that connection, whether it's a moment in front of your altar, contacting someone directly, or journaling/scheduling a moment of gratitude for the people who have helped you get where you are today.

Afterwards, let yourself sit with that feeling of gratitude in your body for as long as you feel comfortable. Then, when you're ready, pick up the tools you identified at the end of the last chapter in "Pour into Practice: Making Time for 'Flow'"—we're going right into flow!

Creativity as a Grounding Tool

Pour into Practice: Enact Your "Flow State Plan!"
It's time to enter flow!

1. Gather your tools, whether for visual art-making, musicking, writing, movement, or whatever terms you devised in "Pour into Practice: Making Time for 'Flow'" for defining what practices were most "flow-accessible" for you.

2. Set them in front of you (whether literally or in your mind), and take a moment to center yourself and get grounded in your body.

3. When you feel grounded, pick up your tools (again, literally or in your mind), and take another moment to (re)ground yourself, with your tools at the ready.

4. When you are ready, you are going to engage in a small, repetitive gesture. You can change the speed or the

direction of your gesture with each repeat, but the size of the gesture itself should not change.

   a. For visual art-making, this might be a single stroke of your tool, repeated over and over again.
   b. For movement or musicking, you might begin with a small movement, a single note, and develop it into a short pattern of movement or sound that you will repeat.

5. Let yourself explore every possible variation that comes to your mind outside of the size of the gesture itself. Eventually, a state of flow should develop, and when you feel that, *then* you can let go of the size of the gesture and allow it to shift. As that last parameter releases, flow into what emerges from there.

6. When you feel a sense of completion, stop to pause and observe whatever may be happening in your body/mind. If what's happening includes an urge to re-enter the flow, go ahead! You may pause and resume as many times as feels meaningful, or stop after the first pause.

Journal anything that feels significant in response to this experience. Then step away from this book and let what you've experienced marinate. Perhaps check in with your accountability buddy to share a bit about what you've learned.

The work will still be here, and you'll be stronger for the break as well!

The exercise above is based on a prompt I (Natasha) received during my PhD studies at Lesley University. It was given during a class taught by Shaun McNiff, though I am not sure if he received the prompt from someone else before him (which is possible). What I appreciate about it, and what may feel meaningful to those experiencing it, is that it takes us back to that first invitation we made to start small and breathe into the possibility of small things becoming larger, deeper, and more meaningful. Every time I embark on this experience, I meet with a different result, and the meaning made is unique, nourishing, and necessary every time.

The space that I take after each creative meaning-making experience is important too. We all need space to imagine in order to sustain the work of healing! And yet, in a society like the United States, where race-based injustice and inequity are ubiquitous and practically constant, space can be hard to find. Reflexivity and solidarity become critical elements in identifying, cultivating, and ensuring the future of spaces, resources, and opportunities where Black people can see and experience surviving and thriving as their whole selves.

We create (and recreate!) the grounds where we can (and must!) re-member ourselves, over and over again, towards wholeness. This is the deeper work of reflexivity, to help us stay grounded in ourselves and in our purposes.

The act of becoming whole/re-establishing wholeness is radical, revolutionary, and critical. In spaces that once declared Black people to be legally 3/5 (three-fifths) of a person, where personhood was denied, where Black bodies were seen as valuable property and Black souls unnecessary accessories, it is vital that Black people get to reclaim the fullness of who we are. We get to re-assert ownership of our bodies, our emotions, our thoughts, and our souls. In a time of continued Anti-Blackness, our healing will be ongoing. We need to choose every day to engage in those practices and actions that affirm our personhood and our divinity.

We can't do any of that in isolation. In the times when I (Adenike) am overwhelmed by the stress and injustice I experience, I am immensely grateful for my Black siblings who rally around me. When they do, I remember that I am part of something bigger, stronger, and more meaningful than just myself.

In many ways, the principle of *ubuntu* is at the core of movements dedicated to social justice and liberation. How can any of us claim to be free when we oppress others, deny them access to resources, and essentially deny their humanity? If others aren't human, how can we be human? Movements for liberation and justice are only successful when they center the needs of the most vulnerable, the most oppressed, and the most disenfranchised.[3] When their voices are amplified, when their input is fully incorporated into plans for restoration and justice, only then do we see real and sustainable change. Here, we dive deeper into the construct of solidarity.

Making Space for Grief and Care

One of the most natural and challenging aspects of solidarity (and reflexivity to some degree as well) is grief. To be among the ranks of the Black, Queer, and disabled is to experience grief frequently, and with complexity. Disability comes for us all, eventually, for as we age, we become disabled, but it comes for people who are most vulnerable with the most intensity. As an example, the COVID-19 pandemic has stolen millions of lives, and yet somehow when information came out that those most susceptible to it were the elderly and disabled, compliance with basic infection control measures decreased, and the risk of infection for disabled people increased.[4] [5] As of this writing, I (Natasha) am less than 30 days from learning of someone new who has either died of, or experienced severe complications from, COVID-19. I spend a lot of time witnessing or experiencing grief.

Grief is another one of those things that comes for us all, but for which not all of us receive the same amount of preparation, like sex ed. It doesn't have to be a monster! Let yourself begin to gently increase your awareness of grief's presence, with care. Though it will, of course, never go away, it will get a little easier each time you make space for it.

Pour into Practice: Developing a Mini-Ritual of Care

As a child, I (Natasha) attended a Catholic school that was right next to a hospital; in particular, it was right next to the landing for the medical helicopters that would occasionally come in. The sound of whirring chopper blades, to this day, urges me in my sixth-grade teacher's voice to stop whatever I am doing and say a quiet prayer for whoever is inside. In recounting this story to my spouse, he told me of his Mexican grandmother doing something similar—stopping to pray for passing ambulances, a practice I have also taken on, though my "prayers" these days are often no more than a deep breath, because sometimes the moment passes quickly and words are scant. Another place I often stop to take a breath of prayer is any time I pass by any sort of police activity, especially if I see anyone Black nearby.

In adopting these practices, no matter how small they may seem, I extend care to myself, or to another person, or a situation, in a ritual way; these are efforts to contribute, however possible, to the highest good of a given moment.

What situations might benefit from you creating similar mini-rituals of care? Your mini-ritual does not have to contain words or any major actions. It can be as simple as: "When I see/experience X, I will take a deep breath."

Whenever you engage in your mini-ritual, make note of any shifts that occur in your body/mind. As you are able, take time to tell someone about what you experienced each time as well. If they feel comfortable, you can invite them to take a breath with you. If this is someone you see or engage with often, maybe this can become an ongoing practice that you share.

Returning to the healing and spiritual practices our Ancestors lived by is one way to do the work of liberation. When we reclaim those values that remind us of our interdependence, that remind us of our interconnectedness with our physical and spiritual worlds, we re-member who we are. We re-member our communities. Living out these principles doesn't mean that other values or philosophies are less important or unnecessary. Living this way helps us make room for more possibilities, for recognizing that my way of being is equally as valid and as necessary as yours. Being in true reciprocal community with each other calls us to find respectful, meaningful ways of working through differences that arise. We understand that our community, our being together, our joint survival, is greater than you or me being right or wrong.

Healing as a way of restoring balance between the physical and the spiritual needs to happen on personal and communal levels. That is how our Ancestors lived. More and more, we see centering our healing, in relationship with others, as a sacred responsibility passed down to us by our African Ancestors. The richness of the traditions they created, the vibrance of their creativity, and the thriving of the societies they created are meant to live on in us and in members of the African Diaspora.

It's ok if we take our time to build these practices up; we just can't give up on healing, or on each other.

Chapter 10

Finding our Wholeness, from the Personal to the Communal

I (Adenike) remember learning a song by The Lettermen in primary school in Trinidad. It was a setting of the quote "No man is an island." Hearing those words at age nine, I didn't think much about them. I think I imagined what it would look like if a person were shaped like a piece of land surrounded by water. Reflecting on them now, I have a sense of how inextricably tied I am to other humans, even when I don't want to know or feel that.

It's funny to think about how we develop as individuals, especially in western society or societies colonized by western countries. When we're infants, our sense of who we are comes from our caregivers. We learn from them and mirror their facial expressions as ways to understand our shared experiences. As children and adolescents, we go to school and are in classes and social groups that continue to shape our sense of who we are and who we think we should be. When we become adults, it seems like things shift a bit. We're focused on developing our careers, building our own families, defining who we are, asserting our autonomy. Sometimes, that can lead us to connect with other similarly minded folks; other times, it can lead us to be more isolated and self-centered.

Graduating college was hard for me, not because I didn't do well academically but because I knew that I would never again be in a space where I'd be living and learning with my friends. The built-in community that college life gave me fell away once I graduated and my friends and I went on our separate journeys. Keeping in touch with occasional phone calls, emails, and now social media isn't quite the same. Being a graduate student didn't bring back that same level of community. I did have more social interactions, as I got to spend time with classmates who became friends as we studied and worked on projects, but they didn't happen as organically since we didn't all live in the same space. As I entered adult life and worked, I found that I had to be more intentional about finding community. There were periods when that was easy, and other times when I was isolated, because who had the time and energy after working to go find friends?

This semi-isolated existence was my norm when I began my doctoral studies. Even though there were more opportunities to engage with similarly-minded people, the underlying reality was that we all had our own lives and our own work to do. Coming together was a rare pleasure. When we were together, I was acutely aware of being the only Black student. I was fortunate to have a Black professor in the program, and I enjoyed working with her and learning about her lived experience in our profession. But aside from her, there was no other student who had a lived understanding of what it meant to be Black and female-identifying in this aspect of our profession. Thankfully, things began to change when I got introduced to another Afro-Caribbean woman also doing doctoral studies in my field at a nearby university. Through connecting with her, I was able to be a founding member of the Black Music Therapy Network, through which I met Natasha.

My experience of being Black in my field led me to do my dissertation on understanding the experiences of Black people as students, clinicians, and educators in music therapy in the United States. Learning about their experiences helped me to make sense of my own and to see that I wasn't as much of an outsider as I thought. It's easy as a Black person to feel like an anomaly in predominantly white spaces. If I never get to connect with other Black people in my field, I remain isolated in some ways, seeing myself as standing apart from the majority. That can lead to having a distorted sense of self and of reality. Being a part of the Black Music Therapy Network and then BCH has helped me re-member who I am and where I come from historically. Our shared Blackness doesn't mean we have lived exactly the same way, but it situates me in a unique context of values, beliefs, practices, and politics. I am no more and no less than my fellow Black music therapists and creatives. We walk different paths along the same road. Coming together reminds me that I am not necessarily the first Black person to see, do, or experience something. Knowing the history of this community of Black music therapists and creatives helps me feel supported, shows me where I can go for guidance, and keeps me from re-inventing the wheel.

Healing and liberation occur on the personal level and communal level. As I become more whole and aligned with those beliefs, values, and practices that promote and sustain my well-being, I naturally become aware of wanting to support well-being in my loved ones and in my communities. I am not an island. I can only get so far in my healing journey on my own. A key part of being whole and well is building and nurturing relationships that sustain me. Humans are social beings. We need to be in relationship with each other for our psychological and spiritual well-being. I think we will never be complete if we don't join with others in healing our communities, in pursuing and creating those conditions that allow us to thrive and be free.

To get to a state of liberation, we must believe unquestionably that our connections to each other, to Blackness, and Blackness itself, are more than beautiful. It is not enough to merely note their existence. If we are all to thrive into the future, we must all believe each other, and ourselves, to be necessary parts of our world. Our Blackness must be necessary—it *is* necessary. Our Blackness is a uniquely powerful, creative way of being in the world. We must love our Blackness. We must love ourselves.

Expanding on the Role Love Plays in Healing Work

Author, feminist theorist, and educator bell hooks noted that the Civil Rights Movement in the United States initially had an ethic of love at its core that guided activism.[1] However, she mourned, that ethic faded as more militant approaches to civil rights gained prominence. In her understanding, despite the gains that were achieved, an essential piece was missing as, generations later, many Black children and adults don't feel loved or believe in love. The absence of love contributes to fractured communities, ongoing wounding, and a lack of shared purpose and vision. hooks said, "To heal our wounded communities, which are diverse and multilayered, we must return to a love ethic, one that is exemplified by the combined forces of care, respect, knowledge, and responsibility."[2] Seeking ways to collectively engage our creativity in our healing and affirming the validity of the worldview and values present in the African Diaspora are acts of love. Through this love, we reclaim our bodies, our souls, our minds, and our power. Through this love, we create our liberation. Love does not eradicate all the ills of the world. Bad days will still come. Awful things will still happen. But love takes us through and lifts us up. It's only fitting to let bell hooks' words speak for themselves here:

> Doing the work of love, we ensure our survival and our triumph over the forces of evil and destruction... [l]ove is our hope and salvation.[3]

Tap in for Reflection: Re-Membering Love

Take a moment to sit with your body and the decision you made to pick up this book and to embark on this journey with yourself, and with us. We're going to call that choice an act of love. What happens in your body when you do this?

In what other ways do you show love for yourself, and for your people? For the planet?

Who can you talk to about this? Make a point to identify that person and make a plan to share some of what you're reflecting on here before going on with your day.

There are many ways that humans show and share love, and each one contributes to the sense of wholeness that each of us feels in our day-to-day lives. And—if we can deepen our intentionality around sharing it—love can be a significant contributor to the sustainability of our work together, towards liberation.

Something that has deeply informed my (Natasha's) understanding of love is raising children. My wonderful spouse and I became parents in 2018, welcoming our second child in late 2023, and the transformative nature of that journey has woken up parts of me that I didn't even know existed. One of those is the part of me capable of cognitive thought after going on seven years of frequently interrupted sleep (ha!), but another significant aspect of myself that "woke up" after becoming a parent is this new dimension of how I experience and express love; it has changed how I steward love within myself, for myself, how my spouse and I steward our love for each other, and the ways in which we are committed to fostering a healthy sense of self-love in others, specifically our children.

This isn't to say that only parents can access deep love, just that this was the route my spirit had to take to access this part of myself. As Sobonfu Some puts it, we are all here to offer some sort of gift to humanity, and all of us have the potential to impact children, whether it's specific children in your life, or future generations in a more general sense![4] Here are some of the ways that my perception and stewardship of love has shifted through my personal crucible of parenthood:

- I see opportunities for love in the seemingly smallest things. Changing a child's diaper, or putting them to sleep, is a deeply vulnerable time. Making space for an extra smile, a song, or some other form of gentleness is a must for me whenever I can, but especially during those times.
- What I extend to my children, I must extend to myself as well. My kids and I talk about what Mama needs, in age-appropriate ways, alongside talking about what they need.
- My immediate nuclear family, while not the only circle of care in my life, is the closest one to my heart, and my sense of wholeness. Whenever my life at large is feeling too big, or out of balance, the path to stability can always be found by coming back to that center.

That last one can be a doozy sometimes. In fact, as a perfect example, just inputting that list above took me multiple trips to the computer, ultimately ending in me putting my youngest on my back and bouncing as I typed, because in 2024 I made the choice to step away from collegiate teaching and work entirely from home as an independent researcher and project director for local and regional community care-based initiatives. This means I'm closer to my kids on a day-to-day, moment-to-moment basis. It also means my kids are closer to my work as well.

Who knows if this is the "right way" to do parenting, but it has been right for me thus far, and, as a dear friend of mine put it recently, another part of this work is for me to be ready for the moment my kids may tell me, after everything I think I've done, that I still missed something or that some choice (or choices!) that I made may have been less helpful than I intended.

Preparing for Rupture and Repair as Natural Parts of the Work

As you work towards finding and sustaining wholeness for yourself and those closest to you, and begin to branch out towards being a whole person working towards liberation with other whole people, you have to be ready to be wrong, and to find yourself in conflict from time to time. This is one of those things that might sound obvious but can be difficult in practice!

Tap in for Reflection: Re-Membering Yourself through Being "Wrong"

How would you describe your relationship with being wrong? Is it something that happens to you often? How accustomed would you say you are to that experience?

Think back to a recent (low stakes, nothing too intense) moment of being wrong. What did you experience in your body the moment you realized that your actions had contributed to what was going on?

Now take a moment to remind your body of the sensation of making something "better" from the first exercise in this book, "Tap in for Refelection: Describe Sensations, Let Memory Support You." Can you feel it? Let yourself deeply remember that feeling.

Now you're going to try and connect the two: that feeling of something getting "better" and the experience of being "wrong." What lives between those two feelings? Maybe this will involve remembering a moment where you made something better after being wrong, or someone helped you to make things better, regardless of who was "wrong." Take a moment to jot down, or maybe even map out, the points of connection from "wrong" to "better" as best you can.

Take breaks if you need to check in with your body and meet its needs before continuing. And don't be afraid to involve other people in this exercise as well, if there's someone you feel the need to consult with for refreshing your memory or taking some other action this experience may motivate you to take.

For a large chunk of my life, I (Adenike) have had a hard time with the idea of being "wrong." Being wrong meant that I messed up, I disappointed others, and I wasn't perfect (forget good enough!). Perfection and people pleasing were huge parts of my relationships with others. It has only been in the last few years that I've been able to truly understand that perfection is a myth. Regardless of my best intentions, I will say or do something that disappoints, offends, hurts, or even harms someone. I don't know and understand everything. Who could? How am I honoring my humanity and that of those around me if I expect complete perfection in all things at all times? In a workshop I attended at the beginning of 2025 led by Dr. Raquel Martin and Dr. Han Ren on becoming an anti-racist and anti-oppressive therapist, they shared about the importance of showing grace to each other as we do the work of justice. They emphasized that the work doesn't call for perfection but for accountability. Once you are aware of the "wrong" you've done, can you acknowledge it and work to make amends? Hearing this encouraged me to work to unlearn and release unrealistic expectations I have of myself and others. We are humans working with other humans. We will mess up. But if we value our community and shared liberation, then we compassionately hold ourselves and each other accountable to living out our values.

Something I (Natasha) was chuckling about with a friend recently was how, since stepping away from full-time teaching, I sometimes miss the feeling of being "existentially bored" in academia, because the experience of regularly facing the deepest parts of myself in community with other folks doing movement work, which makes up more of my day-to-day work now, is hard! When I would be "wrong" in academia, sure, I could have an impact on someone's learning experience, which could be deeply challenging in its own right, but the ways I am "wrong" now have a more immediate and resounding impact on people's material conditions and involve more of my/our sense of self and values in practice. I have spent hours in meetings with people who are deeply committed to the work of healing justice and still struggle to sustain points of connection with each other.

I share this not to be discouraging (though, believe me, sometimes it can feel that way!) but to be real about how difficult and intricate this part of the work can be. Let me use a creative example:

A game that's been a regular part of my life for the past few years has been "I Love Hue," a color-based puzzle game. The player is presented with a gradient of colors, made up of shapes that are then scrambled and have to be reassembled. As I've gotten further into the game, the puzzles have gotten harder in multiple ways: where I would once have to just shift rectangles vertically to make up a fairly straightforward rainbow gradient, I now regularly find myself facing gradients that span maybe only two or three colors in total but contain hundreds of pieces in mixed shape formations. We're talking diamonds, hexagons, triangles, and more, in myriad barely distinguishable shades that have to be moved up, down, or sideways—some that even need to be rotated!—in order to reassemble the gradient. Recently I related to a colleague at one of my community care gigs that playing this game can sometimes remind me of the complexity of healing work; in the beginning, the lines between the version of me that is attempting to heal myself and others around me who have yet to begin that work felt real clear (i.e., "I'm blue but this person is green, so my work goes here and they can stay over there"), but as I progress further in my own journey, alongside people who are also traveling deeper in their own journeys, we are meeting each other at tighter and tighter gradients of our values (i.e., "We're all some kind of greenish blue thing, but my blueish green is different than yours, so now what?"). Sometimes I have to determine whether the lines of distinction we find are such that we can still work together, just keeping the differences between us in mind, or whether we need more distance. Just as surely as seafoam green isn't the same as haint blue, how closely we can work together depends on the context of the puzzle we are trying to solve.

For those moments when I/we want to stay close in community, while holding awareness of our differences, being ready to be wrong and being mindful about the ways we strive to make things better is a way to prepare accountability practices for ourselves, and for our communities. We need those for this work to be sustainable as well.

Pour into Practice: Mapping the Building Blocks of Accountability: Identity, Nourishment, Balance, and Commitment

This exercise will be most meaningful when it is completed by more than two people. Bring some of the folks from your (hopefully) growing pod together to do this with you.

For accessibility purposes, the image is briefly described below, with a short list of the questions/prompts in text-only form. In the accompanying workbook, the questions are also provided with journaling space for those who'd prefer to engage in this exercise in a linear way. You may also wish to craft your own imagery around these questions, and that is welcome as well!

At the end of the image description and questions/prompts list, an enlarged image-based version can be accessed digitally for sharing and printing so you can lay your papers next to each other after filling it out and make even deeper meaning, as the lines of weaving from side to side and top to bottom should form some interesting links!

Here is the image description: Three rectangular patches are laid out vertically over wide bands that weave horizontally across the page. Each patch and band contains prompts and space for writing in responses.

Questions/prompts:

- I AM (you can use any descriptive word (adjective) or noun here):
- I AM NOT:
- Love for myself looks like:
- Love for my people looks like:
- Love from my people looks like:
- This is the kind of (circle one) work/experience/space (or relationship) that nourishes me (this is the place for action words (verbs) or descriptors):
- Why? What happens when I am nourished?
- How? What are the factors that contribute to my nourishment?
- What happens when I am feeling malnourished?
- What are the factors that help me balance my nourishment with other folks' needs?
- Today I commit to:
- My Ancestors remind me:
- I welcome:

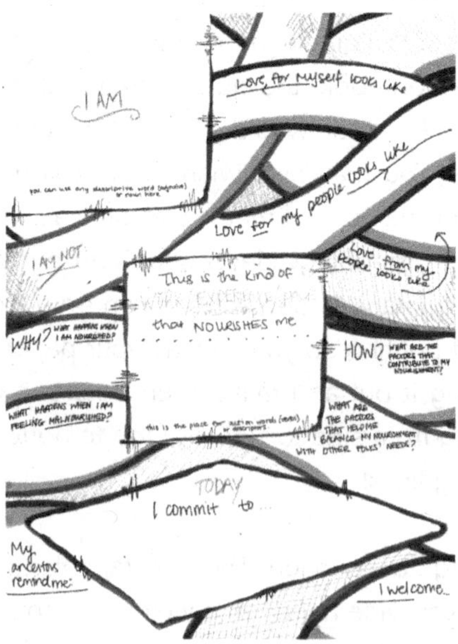

A full-size version of this image can be found in the accompanying workbook.

What we hope this exercise brings out in you and the people you share it with is a sense of deeper connection to, and understanding of, who each of you are, how each of you thrives, and how you can help each other continue to thrive. With that kind of foundation, accountability emerges most naturally and healthily as an extension of care, and never as punishment.[5] Punishment has no place in this structure.[6] The network of relationships you have identified above should all be people and spaces where you are held in accountability, because you are so deeply loved that the people in those spaces want to support you in becoming and sustaining your most whole self, and staying in relationship as you do.

That said, accountability can still feel sticky, and uncomfortable, at times. Resources like Daria Garina's Centered Accountability Mapping course can be helpful with grounding ourselves individually through experiences of conflict and the process of being held in accountability without losing our sense of self or becoming lost in shame spirals. Models like the Creative Interventions Toolkit can also support people looking to move through accountability processes together in community groups.

We also want to be clear in stating how important it is to do this work in a preparatory and reflexive way *before* conflict arises. Similar to how we encouraged you to think about your experiences and processes in relation to pain in Section 2, taking the time for you and the people you are in community with to develop deep understandings of each other and establish shared senses of your values and collective processes for how you want to hold each other in accountability—well before you need to—can help increase the potential for ease and success in the process!

Lifting Off into the Future, and a More Liberated World

These are the "final" touches on building the world we want to see, even though we know this work is never done! We begin within, steeping in our bodies and the Ancestral knowledge we all hold, then extending these threads of knowledge and possibility towards each other, weaving them together with intentionality and care. We pause to make sense and meaning of what we find as we do this, re-integrating "new" Ancestral knowledge into our own bodies and memories, before we reach out to community once more, maybe a little further each time than the last. For example, if there are no Black folks you share mutual trust with who are able complete the final exercise above with you, identify and make a plan to bring yourself one step closer to building that kind of trusting relationship.

And then keep doing it, over and over again.

This is where the work of liberation takes flight.

Throughout this book, we have attempted to steward you, with love, through identifying your personal and Ancestral stake in our world's current state, with particular focus on descendants of the African Diaspora, towards strengthening your own creative tethers to this broader tapestry of life that connects us all. We have opened a portal from which both wounds and possibilities can be seen, both within yourself and between you and your community. Where you go from here is anyone's guess! But we hope and imagine you already see it in your mind's eye, because we have seen ourselves this far. Surely, together, we can see ourselves even further, and even more free.

Section Review

In this section, we started to take the "training wheels" off, so to speak, and look towards the future of building sustainable paths forward for Black-affirming creative healing, including:

- clarifying and affirming the role of ritual in this work
- reviewing our bodies' preferences to determine an entrance point for creative "flow"
- making space for gratitude, grief, and care
- expanding on the role that love plays in healing work
- preparing for rupture and repair as natural parts of the work
- (re)assessing and deepening our practice of entering into creative ritual/play with/in community.

We had fewer reflections and practices in this section than previously in order to allow space for your expanding practices to take their deepest and most sustainable roots. This involved lots of "going back to retrieve it," by reviewing previous reflections and exercises in order to strengthen the threads we have been weaving between Sections 1 and 2:

1. Reflect: Acknowledge Your Rituals, (Re)Assess Associations with Spirituality
    a. Practice: Making Time for "Flow"
2. Practice: Take a Moment to Say Thank You!
    a. Practice: Enact Your "Flow State Plan!"
    b. Practice: Developing a Mini-Ritual of Care
3. Reflect: Re-Membering Love
4. Reflect: Re-Membering Yourself through Being "Wrong"
    a. Practice: Mapping the Building Blocks of Accountability: Identity, Nourishment, Balance, and Commitment

Below is a possible schedule for integrating these practices into your life on a regular basis, infusing them alongside/between the practices recommended in Sections 1 and 2:

Daily	Weekly	Monthly	As you feel led
Describe sensations (from Section 1)	Tend an Ancestral space (from Section 1)	(Re)calculate risks and rewards (from Section 1)	Re(define) your connection to Africa, breathe into what's newly emerging or able to be released (from Section 2)
(Re)ground in your physical environment (from Section 2)	Check in on your Ancestral/bodily connections and tasks (from Section 2): How would you define where you are in your journey right now? What progress are you making? What feels important to make note of or adjust?	(Re)contextualize your experience of pain (or another sensation you can identify and feel led to explore!) (from Section 2)	Poetic (re) construction of any previous exercise (from Section 2): When you look back at what you've constructed, what do you feel led to play with or explore more deeply?

Daily	Weekly	Monthly	As you feel led
Tune into Dreamspace (from Section 1)	Make time for flow at least once per week, more if you've got the space for it!	Revisit your familial/ community context journaling and/or pod-map! (from Section 2)	Enact your mini-ritual of care, however you've defined it, whenever feels right Similarly, remember love and how to hold yourself through experiences of being "wrong"
Make time to say thank you, even if it's just a moment of gratitude at your altar or in your journal!			Revisit your accountability/ identity/ nourishment/ balance and commitment map; continue in conversation/ collaboration with your closest family/community members

Benediction—a Blessing and a Prayer

What we carry is heavy,
heavy as the millions of gallons of water in the Atlantic Ocean,
and heavy as gold that glistens and delights.
Within us are many worlds, many stories, many pasts, many futures.
We are surrounded by our Ancestors' whispers,
their wishes and wails,
their creativity, and their determination;
weaving with fortitude from generation to generation,
we carry, but never alone.
What we carry is not the sum of who we are
as much as it has shaped our journeys.
We can choose what we will continue to carry, what we release,
and what we will take on to help us onwards.
We are lifted by the fires of our spirits,
warm air nourished by our body/mind, knowing:
that as we carry, we are carried too.
We are connected, through the deepening roots of our historical lineages,
and the networks of care we extend to our neighbors;
our branches reaching ever upwards towards the sun,
may we always re-member who we are.
May we always celebrate the wisdom and beauty of our spirits.
May we always find ourselves free and able to see ourselves:
whole.
healed.
healing.
forward.

Pathways: A Shorthand Look at All the Reflections/Practices/Schedules in This Book

From Section 1:

1. Reflect: Describe Sensations, Let Memory Support You
   a. Practice: Calculate Your "Risks and Rewards"

2. Revisit the above exercises as needed!

3. Reflect: Describe Sensations (Again!)

4. Reflect: Revisit Your Memories, Risks, and Rewards

5. Reflect: Identify Your Storyholders
   a. Practice: One Storyholder at a Time

6. Reflect: Assess Your Associations with Spirituality
   a. Practice: Tend to an Ancestral Space
   b. Practice: "Tune In" to Your Dreamspace

7. Reflect: Build Your Own Ancestral Wisdoms List
   a. Practice: Honor Ancestral Wisdom

Below is a possible schedule for integrating these practices into your life on a regular basis:

Daily	Weekly	Monthly	As you feel led
Describe sensations: This can be something you do once a day, in the morning or evening, or at multiple points, with as little/much documentation as you feel led!	Tend an Ancestral space	(Re)calculate risks and rewards: What's coming true? What still feels important? Is there anything that needs to be added or removed?	One storyholder at a time: explore more songs, maybe even build a playlist you listen to occasionally. This can also be paired with tending your Ancestral space!
Tune into your Dreamspace by keeping a journal			

From Section 2:

1. Reflect: Define Your Connection to Africa
    a. Practice: Breathe into Your Connection(s)

2. Reflect: Contextualize Your Experience of Pain
    a. Practice: Poetic (Re)Construction

3. Reflect: Stories of the Inexplicable in Health
    a. Practice: Attune to Your Sense of Bodily Knowing

4. Reflect: Connect the Threads between Our Ancestral and Bodily Knowings
    a. Practice: Prepare to Act on your Connections!

5. Reflect: Sit with the Complexity of Your Ancestral Body's Task

6. Reflect: (Re)Ground in Your Physical Senses and Environment

7. Reflect: Begin to Strategize about Your Familial/Community Environment (and Possible Collaborators on Your Healing Journey!)
   a. Practice: Convert Your Journaling into a Pod-Map!

Below is a possible schedule for integrating these practices into your life on a regular basis:

Daily	Weekly	Monthly	As you feel led
Describe sensations (from Section 1)	Tend an Ancestral space (from Section 1)	(Re)calculate risks and rewards (from Section 1)	Re(define) your connection to Africa, breathe into what's newly emerging or able to be released
Tune into Dreamspace (from section 1)	Check in on your Ancestral/bodily connections and tasks: How would you define where you are in your journey right now? What progress are you making? What feels important to make note of or adjust?	(Re)contextualize your experience of pain (or another sensation you can identify and feel led to explore!)	Poetic (re) construction of any previous exercise: When you look back at what you've constructed, what do you feel led to play with or explore more deeply?

From Section 3:

1. Reflect: Acknowledge Your Rituals, (Re)Assess Associations with Spirituality
   a. Practice: Making Time for "Flow"

2. Practice: Take a Moment to Say Thank You!
   a. Practice: Enact Your "Flow State Plan!"
   b. Practice: Developing a Mini-Ritual of Care

3. Reflect: Re-Membering Love

4. Reflect: Re-Membering Yourself through Being "Wrong"
   a. Practice: Mapping the Building Blocks of Accountability: Identity, Nourishment, Balance, and Commitment

Below is a possible schedule for integrating these practices into your life on a regular basis, infusing them alongside/between the practices recommended in Sections 1 and 2:

Daily	Weekly	Monthly	As you feel led
Describe sensations (from Section 1)	Tend an Ancestral space (from Section 1)	(Re)calculate risks and rewards (from Section 1)	Re(define) your connection to Africa, breathe into what's newly emerging or able to be released (from Section 2)
(Re)ground in your physical environment (from Section 2)	Check in on your Ancestral/bodily connections and tasks (from Section 2): How would you define where you are in your journey right now? What progress are you making? What feels important to make note of or adjust?	(Re) contextualize your experience of pain (or another sensation you can identify and feel led to explore!) (from Section 2)	Poetic (re) construction of any previous exercise (from Section 2): When you look back at what you've constructed, what do you feel led to play with or explore more deeply?
Tune into Dreamspace (from Section 1)	Make time for flow at least once per week, more if you've got the space for it!	Revisit your familial/ community context journaling and/ or pod-map! (from Section 2)	Enact your mini-ritual of care, however you've defined it, whenever feels right Similarly, remember love and how to hold yourself through experiences of being "wrong"
Make time to say thank you, even if it's just a moment of gratitude at your altar or in your journal!			Revisit your accountability/ identity/nourishment/ balance and commitment map; continue in conversation/ collaboration with your closest family/ community members

The Workbook

Supplemental Pages for Working through the Reflection/Practice Prompts

SECTION 1

TAP IN FOR REFLECTION: DESCRIBE SENSATIONS, LET MEMORY SUPPORT YOU

Take a moment to name a **sensation** you feel in your body right now. This is different than an emotion. This is something to do with the way your **body** feels. It may be something that **informs** your emotions, but this is the thing that comes **before** your brain begins to interpret.

You can explore the sensation coming to your brain with your mind alone, or with a pen and paper. Words like "tired" may come to your mind first, or "tension"; any of that is ok! Whatever word you arrive at, write it down.

Now we're going to go deeper. Within any given word there are additional qualities worth excavating, because your definition of "tired" or "tense" may not be the same as someone else's. What is "tired" to you? Is it a heaviness in your eyelids or something you feel in other parts of your body? If you named "tension," where is it? Does it have a specific point of origin, or does it feel widespread? Is it a high level of tension or something you can release just by bringing awareness to it? This is the level of **specificity** we want to encourage here.

Once you've written your word, and added some specificity to its description, take a breath or two before going any further.

Can you remember another time you felt this way? Let yourself lightly explore the memory of the feeling, just for a moment. Let it be like a hologram around you, lightly projecting out of the corner of your eye, easy to disperse at will, otherwise immersive. A memory you can pause, rewind, or blow away. If you feel so led, describe it here.

Now shift your focus to an experience following that feeling—one where something (or someone) improved what you were experiencing, at any time, in a meaningful way. Let your senses lean in to that memory of **meaning**. What was happening to your skin, in response to the temperature, or other people or objects about you, wherever you were in that moment? What did the air smell like?

Take a moment to let this memory give you a message. As with most gifts, you don't really get to choose what you will receive. This message will be chosen for you as whatever thought first enters your head after you finish this sentence…

Whether this message came from your subconscious, the Holy Spirit, an Ancestor, or the most recent food to enter your digestive system, you will know this message to be unique to this moment. Sit with this moment; as you do this, know that if this feels hard or uncomfortable in any way, it is ok to stop, try again later, or move on. **You know your body/mind best** and can trust it to signal to you when it's time to change gears, in any direction.

Ok?

If/when you feel ready, let the message you received just now simmer within you for a bit. Play it back in your memory or read it aloud as many times as feels necessary for you to commit it to memory, such that it can autoplay in your mind while you feel deeper into your body. Set a timer if you feel the need to contain the experience in some way. Again, you know your body/mind best. **Pay attention** to what happens within you as the message simmers.

Describe/display your gift, as you feel led, below.

What does your breath feel like right now? What else might be happening in your body right now? And how might it relate to the sensation you made note of earlier?

Take a moment to jot down anything that has shifted in your body in response to this experience. Then, **step away** from this book for a time. Go for a walk, get a drink of water or some food to eat, and let what you've experienced marinate. The work will still be here when you get back, and you'll be better equipped on the other side of a break.

POUR INTO PRACTICE: CALCULATE YOUR "RISKS AND REWARDS"

What are the risks of healing for you? What are the potential rewards? List them below.

Risks of healing (things you may need to work through or let go of):	**Potential rewards:**

Remember, take your time with this. Some responses may arrive quickly and with great clarity. Others may emerge more slowly (if at all), and with more nuance and gray areas. It's all possible!

Now let's bring in some creativity!

Remember, perfection is not the point. Our Ancestors were creative, and so are you. Creativity can begin with the simplest of actions. For this moment, let's focus on a short series of choices. You will want to have some colored pens/pencils, crayons, or markers near you for this:

1. Identify one word from each of the columns you have created: one risk and one reward.

One risk:	**One reward:**

2. Center your focus on the risk you have chosen. You are going to ask yourself a question about that word. The question is not about what the word means in any literal sense. The question is going to be about choosing a symbol to represent that word.
3. The symbol you choose is going to be a color or a texture. When you look at the risk you have chosen, what color or texture rises in your mind? Let the color/texture become vibrantly clear in your mind. It might help you to say your word, color, or texture aloud as you sit with it.

Color/texture associated with your risk:

4. Place that color or texture next to the word it represents in your list. You may wish to outline or highlight your word in the color you chose, or make some other representation, like a wavy or jagged line to indicate texture. Remember, your symbol does not have to be perfect! You are simply making a choice to make meaning in some small way. This is a creative act!

Risk:	**Color/texture:**

5. When you have completed the representation of your symbol next to your risk word, repeat this series of actions/choices for the word you've chosen on your rewards list.

Reward:	**Color/texture:**

6. Afterwards, sit for a minute or two with any feelings that may have arisen for you as you chose these symbols. You may wish to journal these feelings, sit with them further, or breathe them out and go on with your day. Any/all of these feelings and decisions are ok! Recognize them and let them flow as they will, without judgment.

Note: There are many ways this experience can be adapted. You may wish to try out other kinds of symbols, like sound or gesture. Whatever you choose, resist the urge to create something complicated or lengthy. Let it be simple; let it be small, like spelling out the letters of your risk or reward in its color/texture, focusing closely on every stroke, every little detail that you make. Let yourself find satisfaction in the infinite potential of one choice at a time.

TAP IN FOR REFLECTION: DESCRIBE SENSATIONS (AGAIN!)

Check in with your body. Make note of any sensations that feel important to name, or to address.

If you're feeling tension, take a moment to breathe or stretch. If you're feeling hungry or thirsty, or tired, meet those needs as best you can before moving ahead.

TAP IN FOR REFLECTION: REVISIT YOUR MEMORIES, RISKS AND REWARDS

Check in with your body again, making note of any sensations and meeting any needs.

Now revisit that memory of meaning from the reflection where we first invited you to describe sensations, "Tap in for Reflection: Describe Sensations, Let Memory Support You" and remember a time when someone or something improved the situation you were in, in some way.

Take a moment to recall the sensations of the meaning you made (any scents, sounds, etc.) as you revisit that memory and the memory of the message you received from it. You can rewrite the message or any relevant reminders for yourself here as needed.

Consider the possible value in the meaning that the Weavers (the family centered in the vignettes of Chapter 2) are making on their trip (with the photos they're taking, stories they're telling, physical interactions they are having, etc.).

What value might that meaning be having on their bodies in these first few days? What value might you imagine that it holds for them down the road, years later? Generations later?

Now take a moment to revisit your own list of risks and rewards in relation to your personal healing journey, and update the rewards list with anything you've named above that you hadn't previously listed there. Or, if you want, you can rewrite the whole list here.

Risks of healing (things you may need to work through or let go of):	**Potential rewards:**

Check in with your body once again, and take another break, if need be.

Hopefully, each time you do this, the transitions between checking in, naming sensations, making meaning, and documenting what emerges are beginning to feel smoother and more easeful to do. If not, that's ok! And if it feels like any changes you're experiencing are incremental, that's ok too! In fact, that's probably for the best—remember, small, incremental changes are more sustainable. Continue to be patient with yourself!

TAP IN FOR REFLECTION: IDENTIFY YOUR STORYHOLDERS

Consider: Who are the people, blood-related or not, who hold and share the stories of who "we" are in your family? Write their names in this space.

After you have populated your list, allow your hands to simply sit on the page and—as your comfort/capability allows—read the names slowly, aloud. If that doesn't feel possible for you right now, that's ok! You may consider simply going forward into your week and just paying attention to anything in your environment or history that might draw one or more of these people forward into your mind. Make particular note of anything that happens in your body (tightness/relaxation, any additional urges or emotions, etc.) anytime this happens.

POUR INTO PRACTICE: ONCE STORYHOLDER AT A TIME

When you are ready (as in, when you feel comfortable enough to sit with your list), you are going to choose one of the people or stories that you've identified and find a song to accompany some deeper reflection. Here, we're going to recommend that you go with a person or story that is relatively "low stakes," that is, someone who doesn't stir up feelings that are too deep or strong. They may have been someone who barely made your list, but something in you just knew they had to be there. Song identification is going to be part of how you explore the reason why you knew this. Here are the steps to this process:

1. Write the name/title of the person or story you've selected below or on a fresh, blank sheet of paper, separate from the list you built previously.

2. Open your platform of choice: you may have a subscription to Apple Music that will make this easier for you. If not, or if you'd rather have videos to work with, you can use YouTube.

3. Sit with the name/title you've written, and ask yourself: When I think about this person/story, what sounds, instruments, songs, or artists come to my mind?

Person/story:	Song/instruments:

   a. If a song comes to your mind right away, hit play!
   b. If a song doesn't come to your mind right away, that's ok! You can google "songs with..." and insert any sounds or instruments that come to mind, or sift through the discography of any artist that comes to mind, to help you gradually narrow down to something that feels right.

4. Take your time! Listen to any songs in their entirety if you can, and don't be afraid to take breaks in this process to let things sit and come back to the list at alternate days/times if need be.
   a. As you sit with whatever song you ultimately choose, look at the name/title you've written down and think back to the earlier color/texture exercise, "Pour into Practice: Calculate Your 'Risks and Rewards.'" Is there a color or texture you'd assign to this person/story along with this song? Or anything else that comes to your body/mind that is worth noting?
   b. Document whatever comes up, whether it is a color/texture or other thought or feeling. Even an urge can be noted with

a phrase like, "Thinking about this person/story makes me want to..."

Person/story:	**Song/instruments:**	**Color/texture/thought/ feeling:**

5. While you're documenting, resist any urge to build a whole playlist or write beyond a single page at this time—we can do any/all of that later. This is still the time to keep things "small" and allow things to expand from there without pressure.
    a. If you want to save a song to access later, you can "like" it in YouTube or save it to your general library in Apple Music.
    b. If you feel like you want to explore/work through more thoughts/ feelings on this story or person, take those thoughts/feelings to someone you trust and start a conversation! If the person/ story you thought of is/has a source you can still access easily, maybe you could share the song you chose with them.

6. Breathe through anything that emerges from this experience, without judgment. Check in with your body and meet any needs (hunger, thirst, fatigue) that you may sense, before going on with your day.

TAP IN FOR REFLECTION: ASSESS YOUR ASSOCIATIONS WITH SPIRITUALITY

What happens in your body when you consider the idea of spirituality as being part of a healing practice? Make note of any tension or release that occurs in your body.

Now allow yourself to briefly consider what might be behind it. Are there messages or stories associated with any of your current sensations? Make shorthand/surface-level notes of those messages or stories as well, not to dive too deeply into them now but just as a temperature check on how this topic lands in your body/mind at this time.

Whatever emerges, breathe through it, and remember that beautiful thing about creativity and knowledge: there is always room for nuance, possibility, and difference of perspective between people, and across time!

POUR INTO PRACTICE: TEND TO AN ANCESTRAL SPACE

Altar tending can be an incredibly nourishing creative and healing practice. As we mentioned, you may already have one or more altar spaces (or something like it, if you'd rather call it/them something else) in your home! Take a moment to think of any space where you have collected images of, or items from, people who were significant to your life and are no longer living. Identify it below.

How might you tend to that space today? Perhaps it's something as simple as dusting a picture frame or bookshelf, or picking up a book or other item of significance to that person and holding it in your hands for a moment while you think of them.

If you don't have an altar(like) space in your home, perhaps you might build one. Start with just one image or item at a time. Set it somewhere significant, and let time pass as you tend to it, adding or expanding the space only as it feels natural to do so. If the person you are honoring was someone on the list you built in "Pour into Practice: One Storyholder at a Time," maybe you might play the song you identified for them as you build or tend. Natasha actually has a practice of singing songs of personal significance to each of the Ancestors on her altar anytime she tends to that space!

Altar items:	**Practices:**

Make note of any sensations or emotions that may arise for you as you take the time to tend to your beloved images or items, without judgment. Meet any bodily or emotional needs that may arise: eat, sleep, cry, or find someone to talk to.

Emerging sensations/emotions, etc.:	**How I'm tending to them:**

Return to this practice, and the documentation of it, periodically, to keep it up to date. At this point, there may be emerging evidence of how thoughts/feelings within you may be changing over time. These do not have to be major shifts; in fact, you may not even find yourself shifting in any discernible way other than that you are taking more time to sit with things than you were before. But even that is important, and worth noting!

POUR INTO PRACTICE: "TUNE IN" TO YOUR DREAMSPACE

Having a dream is just one more possible step of bridging the physical and the spiritual. Next steps might include remembering the dream and reflecting on the message within it, whether through journaling or speaking with someone about the dream after the fact. Natasha has even utilized a practice in the past of writing short stories based on dreams!

To strengthen your connection to the spiritual through dreams, it might help you to develop specific pre-sleep rituals, like the setting of intentions and avoiding screens for at least 30 minutes prior to sleep. Keeping a dream journal beside your bed will make it easier to record your dreams upon waking, when your memory of them is at its freshest. You could also use the voice memo function of your cell phone or other recording device to recall your dream.

My pre-sleep dream ritual:

Reviewing what you've written or recorded on your own, shaping it into a short story, or discussing it with someone whose counsel you trust later in the day/week/month might give you insight into what you could do (or need to do!) in response to your dream.

My post-waking process for documenting dreams:

TAP IN FOR REFLECTION: BUILD YOUR OWN ANCESTRAL WISDOMS LIST

What are your Ancestral Wisdoms around healing? These can be words a family member has said that you hold close whenever you are going through a difficult time, meals that have nourished your soul, or other practices that you have observed being passed down through your family; everything from cold remedies to how you tend to each other during rituals like the birth of a child or death of a loved one is fair game!

Ancestral Wisdoms—a personal list:

POUR INTO PRACTICE: HONOR ANCESTRAL WISDOM

1. Consider any symbols (images/items, songs, scents, etc.) that come to your mind with any of the stories you've listed above.

2. Doodle your symbol next to the Ancestral Wisdom you associate them with. For instance, if cinnamon is part of a recipe you remember, you might doodle a little cinnamon stick next to that Ancestral Wisdom on your list.

Ancestral Wisdom:	**Doodle:**

3. Check in with your body and pause to meet any needs that may arise as you do so (for food, rest, etc.).

4. Go on with your day if need be, *or*, if you want to take this even further, after you've added your doodles, you might proceed into building a digital or physical collage from magazines or pictures you find online that match (or relate to) what you've doodled, bringing them together in some meaningful way.

Consider as you do so: how might those stories and actions affirm and challenge us to live more fully into our wholeness?

SECTION 2:

TAP IN FOR REFLECTION: DEFINE YOUR CONNECTION TO AFRICA

Read the following poetic affirmation, and asses your body as you do so.

> *"I see Africa in you, and I honor it.*
> *Whether it is blood that runs through your veins,*
> *or blood that your Ancestors have touched.*
> *I call it Mother.*
> *Tell me where your Ancestors come from.*
> *Here is the African in me: she is old, gray,*
> *full of wisdom and wit.*
> *And pain too.*
> *All of life has been her teacher.*
> *What might we learn from each other?*
> *What meaning might we make from this Blood of the Mother?"*

Check in with your body for a moment: how are you feeling? Is there tension anywhere that you might need to release? How's your breath? Your hunger or energy levels?

What actions might you need to take right now to meet any needs identified above? This could include taking in some extra oxygen, feeding yourself, or drinking some water.

POUR INTO PRACTICE: BREATHE INTO YOUR CONNECTION(S)

This is going to be our first official invitation to use your body, beyond writing something down or taking a deep breath. You are going to develop a small movement or gesture. We recognize that moving our bodies may feel strange or uncomfortable for some people, so we are going to intentionally keep this small, and again, remember, you are in control! If something feels like it pushes beyond the realm of reasonable discomfort for you, stop and reset. There is time, and there are many paths we might take. Work with what works for you.

1. Ask yourself: What is my **connection** to the African continent? In what way(s) does that connection manifest?
   a. Maybe it is blood, as the poem above mentions, or maybe you know a story of your family that connects you in history, or maybe the connection is just the world we live in now and the Black folks who occupy the spaces in which you live and work.

   b. Take a moment to just sit with your answer.

2. Now ask yourself: If I were to **imagine** that connection as something **tangible**, what would it be? A piece of string? A strand in a web? A wave in the ocean? Where in my body does that string/strand/wave connect? And what does that feel like?
   a. The question of how something "feels" may lead you into an intellectual answer: resist this! You want to feel into your body in a literal way. This may mean bringing one or both of your hands to a point in your body where a string/strand/wave might touch you, and imagining the sensation of such an object/texture.
   b. Breathe into the feeling, and *then* you can write the feeling down.

3. Return to your body. When you feel as though you have a grasp of how your connection to Africa feels in your body, take a deep breath, and as you exhale, let your body make some small movement or gesture—just for a moment!—in response to that connection.
   a. This is your Connection Gesture, and it could be as small as the breath itself, or you may need to take a second or third breath before a movement comes. Let instinct guide you!

i. Examples: If you've conceptualized a string or a strand, maybe your hands grasp that string/strand and pull, ever so slightly. Or if you've imagined a wave, your body might rock forward and backward slightly.

b. Whatever it is, if you feel comfortable with this small movement, repeat it a few times. If not, just let the movement moment pass and breathe into stillness afterwards. When you are ready, describe your gesture here.

c. Take note of how the feeling of engaging with that connecting sensation might settle or move through your body or emotions.

4. Meet any needs that might arise from this point, including creative needs! If you are a natural mover or a dancer, go ahead and put on a piece of music (maybe even the piece you chose earlier in "Pour into Practice: One Storyholder at a Time" to represent a person/story in your family!) and let your body move even further. Or maybe you need to show this movement to someone else. Or maybe none of this applies to you, and you just need to think about all this for a while before you can move forward into your day or whatever comes next. It's all possible, and only you know what's best for you.

How I'm tending to my needs in this moment:

5. Breathe.

TAP IN FOR REFLECTION: CONTEXTUALIZE YOUR EXPERIENCE OF PAIN

Who in your life do you talk to about pain (whether physical, emotional, or otherwise), other than doctors or related health professionals? Where do those conversations happen? And how do you talk about pain with those people/in those spaces? Begin to make note of the descriptive adjectives you use to describe your pain. Below is an example from Natasha. Your own table might look similar, or different.

***Who* I talk to about pain**	***Where* those conversations happen**	***How* I describe my pain**
Example: My spouse/ family **My experience:**	Example: At home, in phone (audio/video/text) communications **My experience:**	Example: Cramping, tightness, draining **My experience:**

POUR INTO PRACTICE: POETIC (RE)CONSTRUCTION

Look at your list of how you describe pain. Read it like a poem. As you do so, allow yourself to take some creative liberties—maybe move a punctuation mark around or move some words onto a new line. As you make each change, pause and sit with what you're creating, looking at the words like they're a piece of visual art. Do they look the way you want them to? You can use the space below to rewrite anything as you feel led.

Allow yourself to play with even the most fundamental "rules" of grammar or spelling. You have that power! And as you do this, ask yourself: What other power might I have? What else might I be able to shift, in even the smallest of ways? Here's a little more space for play, if you'd like.

TAP IN FOR REFLECTION: STORIES OF THE INEXPLICABLE IN HEALTH

Many individuals have family stories of seemingly impossible occurrences in their family's health history. Some may call these miracles, while others simply acknowledge them as "luck" or synchronicity. These may be stories that you've been encouraged to hide in the past, or only tell to certain people, like someone coming back from the brink of death, or opening their eyes in the moment before departure from life, right after hearing a prayer or song that held meaning for them. Sometimes these moments are among our most precious memories. Take some time to document one such story from your family. As you do, take note of what happens in your body/mind, and meet any needs that may arise—to feed yourself, rest, or reach out to a loved one—before moving on to the rest of this chapter.

My/family story:	**Space for noting anything happening in my body/ mind:**

POUR INTO PRACTICE: ATTUNE TO YOUR SENSE OF BODILY KNOWING

We're jumping straight to the art on this one!

You're going to be trying an adaptation of "Somatic Self-Portraits," a Creative Body-Scanning exercise that I (Natasha) first had the gift of experiencing from Ellen Bartel during a conference gathering of the International Somatic Movement Education and Therapy Association (ISMETA). This is what you will need:

- Your body, fed and well rested, or as close to those as you can get it!
- A piece of paper (or there is a blank space at the end of this exercise if you prefer).
  - Any kind will do, but if you want to spring for cardstock or something with similar thickness, that might be beneficial.
- Something to write/draw with.
  - Ideally this will be a tool that won't bleed through the paper or struggle with an uneven surface (because you won't be working with a table or anything super firm to press on!). I recommend a gel pen or a non-mechanical pencil.
  - If you have thicker paper, a marker would probably be fine, and may in fact yield the clearest results!
- Time: at least ten minutes.
  - You can set a timer for the first five minutes or listen to a song of that length while you work.

Please note that this is an exercise that is going to invite you to "scan" your body with your mind's eye, from top to bottom, and then move your hand/tool with this scan in mind. This is something that people may have varying degrees of challenge or comfort with. Remember, only you know your limits, when you are in a space to be challenged, and when a challenge might actually be unsafe for you to engage with. Move forward only at the pace of your own capacity, with care.

Here's exactly what you'll be doing with those tools:

1. Hold the paper up to your chest with one hand and your tool in the other.
   a. Let whatever hand is holding the paper be in contact with both the paper and your body.
   b. Let whichever hand is holding your tool rest gently on your lap for now.

2. Breathe. Feel the paper and your hand rising and falling, in time.

3. Close your eyes. Let your mind center in on the top of your head, imagining a sensor just above it, gently collecting data.
   a. You are in charge of that sensor, its movement, and how much data it collects.

4. When you're ready, imagine that sensor moving downward from the top of your head to the tips of your toes. As it moves, bring your tool hand up and place the tip of the tool to the paper.

5. On your next exhale, begin to move the tool to draw a representation of your body from top to bottom, as perceived by the sensor you are controlling: in response to the signals that sensor is giving you.
   a. An example of this can be found in this TikTok video I recorded of myself doing this exercise in 2021: www.tiktok.com/@blackcreativehealing/video/6937759473989717253
   b. Your drawing will not be literal in any sort of "photorealistic" way. Resist the urge to be "certain" of whether what you're drawing looks anatomically correct or aesthetically pleasing. Whether the thing "makes sense" in a visual way is not the point. You are responding to sensations in your body first. You can look later.
      i. Example: Feeling tension anywhere? Breathe, notice it, then

let your tool hand move in whatever way that sensation has motivated your hand to!

ii. Moving in response to your body's sensations may result in tapping or dragging your tool against/across the paper on your chest in patterns that may or may not resemble anything visually, and that's ok. Just work your way through your body, and the paper, from top to bottom, interpreting each sensation with your tool.

6. When you have reached the bottom of your body, or your paper (whichever happens first), stop. Breathe. Thank your body for the messages you are about to interpret.

7. When you are ready, turn your paper around and look at it.
   a. What do you feel when you look at it?

   b. How would you describe what you see and what you feel in response, i.e., when you look at a certain marking you made with your tool, can you tell what sensation you were responding to?
   c. If you feel so led, write your description(s) down (so you can reference them later!).

Description:	Sensation it refers to:

d. Now: take a moment to explore what might be in between what you see and how you feel. This might be through more writing, finding additional words to flesh your descriptions out, or leveraging your body in a way similar to the exercise "Tap in for Reflection: Define Your Connection to Africa," letting movement be your tool for interpretation for those bits of connective tissue between your feelings and thoughts.

What is emerging as I continue exploring:

e. You may not feel led to do anything more than sit with what you feel when you look at the paper—and that's ok too! In the coming sections, we're going to go deeper with our creative choices and actions, but this is one last moment to just sit with the top layer of what you are sensing and experiencing.

8. Save your portrait somewhere safe (because we may return to it later!) and go on with your day, with gentle attention to your body's needs—keep it as hydrated/fed/rested as possible!

My Somatic Portrait (insert your piece of paper here, or use this page for the exercise itself!).

TAP IN FOR REFLECTION: CONNECT THE THREADS BETWEEN OUR ANCESTRAL AND BODILY KNOWINGS

It's time to begin getting really clear about the throughlines we've identified thus far. We're going to take this time to look back at the first two sections of this book and identify some spaces/resources we will need to consult for the final section to come.

1. Go back to your answers from the exercise "Tap in for Reflection: Build Your Own Ancestral Wisdoms List," in Section 1, Chapter 4. Make note of any Ancestral Wisdoms relating to natural remedies (foods, herbs, etc.) or other healing practices (praying, grief rituals, etc.).

2. Now find the exercise "Pour into Practice: Breathe into Your Connection(s)" from Section 2, Chapter 5. Revisit the Connection Gesture you arrived at for representing your connection to the Motherland, and write a brief description of it below.

a. If you were someone who chose to put on a piece of music and dance, record yourself doing it again, then view the video and write down brief/basic descriptions of any moments that stand out to you. Or if you showed this movement to someone else, go back to that person and ask them to describe what they remember of the movement and/or conversation about it, and write down whatever stands out to you from that moment of recollection.

3. Ask yourself: What lives between what I've written about my Ancestral Wisdoms and what I've written about my connection to Africa?
   a. You may identify feelings you have/had that are similar in both exercises, or common words/themes you used in your responses, or you may see no connection whatsoever. Either way, this is data you can use!

i. If you identify common feelings, words, or themes, find a way to identify and/or tie them together, either by highlighting them all in the same color or literally drawing a line between them.
ii. If you see no connection whatsoever, write this down: "I do not yet see a thread between my Ancestral Wisdoms and what I have written of my connection to Africa." That word—"yet"—is important, because we aim to remedy the situation around it!

POUR INTO PRACTICE: PREPARE TO ACT ON YOUR CONNECTIONS!

1. Whether you identified a connection in the above reflection exercise or not, you're going to write a declarative sentence about what your Ancestral Body knows.
   a. My in-chapter example merges my Ancestral Wisdom with my Connection Gesture, reading: "My Ancestral Body knows many ways to stay alive." Yours might do the same, or...
   b. ...if you couldn't identify a connection, or the connection you identified doesn't easily fit into the sentence structure we've invited above, you can craft your defining statement from either the Ancestral Wisdom or the Connection Gesture that you identified, because both of those things are knowledges held by your body today!

2. Now, you are going to craft this knowledge statement into a task—a sort of "next step" to undertake. To help you get there, you're going to use the following formulaic sentence: "I want to learn more about the ways my Ancestors ...."

a. As an example, my task might read: "I want to learn more about the ways my Ancestors stayed alive."

b. Read your task back to yourself and feel how your body reacts. For me, I feel my head sort of cocking to one side like, "That doesn't read quite the way I want it to." You can follow those kinds of signals! With a little tweaking, I've revised my task to: "I want to learn more about the ways my Ancestors sustained themselves."

It is important to note here that the task you assign for yourself may lead you into more complicated places, like wanting to know more about your Ancestors' responsibility for certain atrocities, or you may find yourself articulating a task that leads you to somewhere further away from Africa; all of that is ok in this moment! Whether or not your thread brings you closer to the continent in the ways you want or expect, you have just articulated a path towards strengthening a thread of connection that you either didn't have before or couldn't clearly articulate until this moment invited you to do so. You are already on your way to making the tapestry of your lineage stronger. So remember, if something has not been uncovered or healed (yet!), it doesn't mean it can't be uncovered or healed later! All things in their time.

TAP IN FOR REFLECTION: SIT WITH THE COMPLEXITY OF YOUR ANCESTRAL BODY'S TASK

1. Find a place and time where you can sit comfortably. Take a moment to get tuned in to your environment and your breath, without judgment. Just notice the sights, sounds, and cadences of your body in this moment.

2. Close your eyes and do a brief scan of your body, similar to the "Somatic Self-Portraits" exercise in "Pour into Practice: Attune to Your Sense of Bodily Knowing" but without the writing/drawing tools, just making note of any tension or other state of being in your body that feels important to track.

3. Find and reread the task you identified for yourself in "Pour into Practice: Prepare to Act on your Connections!" As you read it, pay attention to your body, and anything that may shift or respond to reviewing your task.
    a. For reference, the one I (Natasha) had identified for myself was: "I want to learn more about the ways my Ancestors sustained themselves."
    b. Make note of anything that shifts or changes.

4. You're going to turn any noted shifts or changes into subtasks for yourself. Take a moment to reformulate them as such by adding a phrase like: "I want to know more about this shift that happens when I think about my task."
   a. If you didn't note any shifts, that's still data you can track! You can note: "I want to know more about the lack of shifts I feel when I think about my task."

5. Also consider any prerequisite or clarifying actions that your task may require. For instance, in order for me to know more about the way my Ancestors sustained themselves, I need to know who my Ancestors were and what part(s) of the world they were situated in. Finding out who my Ancestors were may require speaking to specific people or looking up/subscribing to a service to help me on my way. Each of those needs is a new task, yielding new information that will then require processing into additional tasks, like identifying a specific group of Ancestors to focus my attention on rather than trying to take them all on at once.

In order for me to:
I might need to:

a. As you note each of these prerequisites or clarifying actions, do additional scans to catch any extra shifts or changes that may be needed to add to your (hopefully) growing list of subtasks. Here is some space for noting anything else that may be emerging.

TAP IN FOR REFLECTION: (RE)GROUND IN YOUR PHYSICAL SENSES AND ENVIRONMENT

Feel your feet planted on the floor or supported by what you're sitting or resting on. Touch what's beside you, like a table, pillow, or the floor. Inhale slowly and deeply. Exhale slowly and completely. Notice three objects in the room you're in, and name them out loud, or write them below.

TAP IN FOR REFLECTION: BEGIN TO STRATEGIZE ABOUT YOUR FAMILIAL/ COMMUNITY ENVIRONMENT (AND POSSIBLE COLLABORATORS ON YOUR HEALING JOURNEY!)

Take some time to journal on the following prompts:

- How do you generally engage as a member of your family and/or community with other family/community members?

  - Is this how you want/choose to engage? If so, describe some elements of what you do that you want to ensure you keep doing. If not, that's ok, just sit with that awareness.

- What are some patterns that you see repeating over and over again in your family/community, whether they are patterns of behavior or things that seem to follow or keep happening? Pay particular attention to any patterns that may cause difficulty for your family/community, pausing to reground in your physical environment, and be gentle with yourself as needed!

  - Identify what elements of those patterns you can control. What might be necessary for you to do or change so that you don't perpetuate patterns of harm within your family/community?

- Who can you share this with in your family/community at this time, in order to invite them to walk beside you in a collaborative healing journey?
  - If you can't identify anyone who would be safe for you to do this with at this time, who might be safe for you to do this with in the future, if you were able to build a little more trust? Or

is this something that you might need to reach outside your immediate family/community to connect with someone over?

- How else might you learn what is needed for your family/community to recover from harm?

- Anyone else (whether a person or an organization) you can partner with?

POUR INTO PRACTICE: CONVERT YOUR JOURNALING INTO A POD-MAP!

A template crafted by Natasha sits on the next page.

In the center of the image, a circle with a little curl above it is meant to hold your name, with solid spirals surrounding it. Those are intended for the names of those people or orgs closest to you in trusting relationship. These may or may not be people or orgs that live or operate physically close to you, but you may wish to make different maps to distinguish your "neighborhood" pod from other collections of people/orgs.

Encircling all the solid spirals are circles framed with dashed lines. Those indicate people or orgs who may need more trust or time to feel more firmly connected. Along the edges of the image are curved lines, dashes, and squiggles forming a border. The different textures in those lines/dashes/squiggles are not just aesthetic in nature but can also be used as suggestions for lines you can draw between circles to indicate the different ways each one may be connected to you (blood relatives, neighbors, friends, etc.). Of course, you can also create your own textures and keys for this map as well!

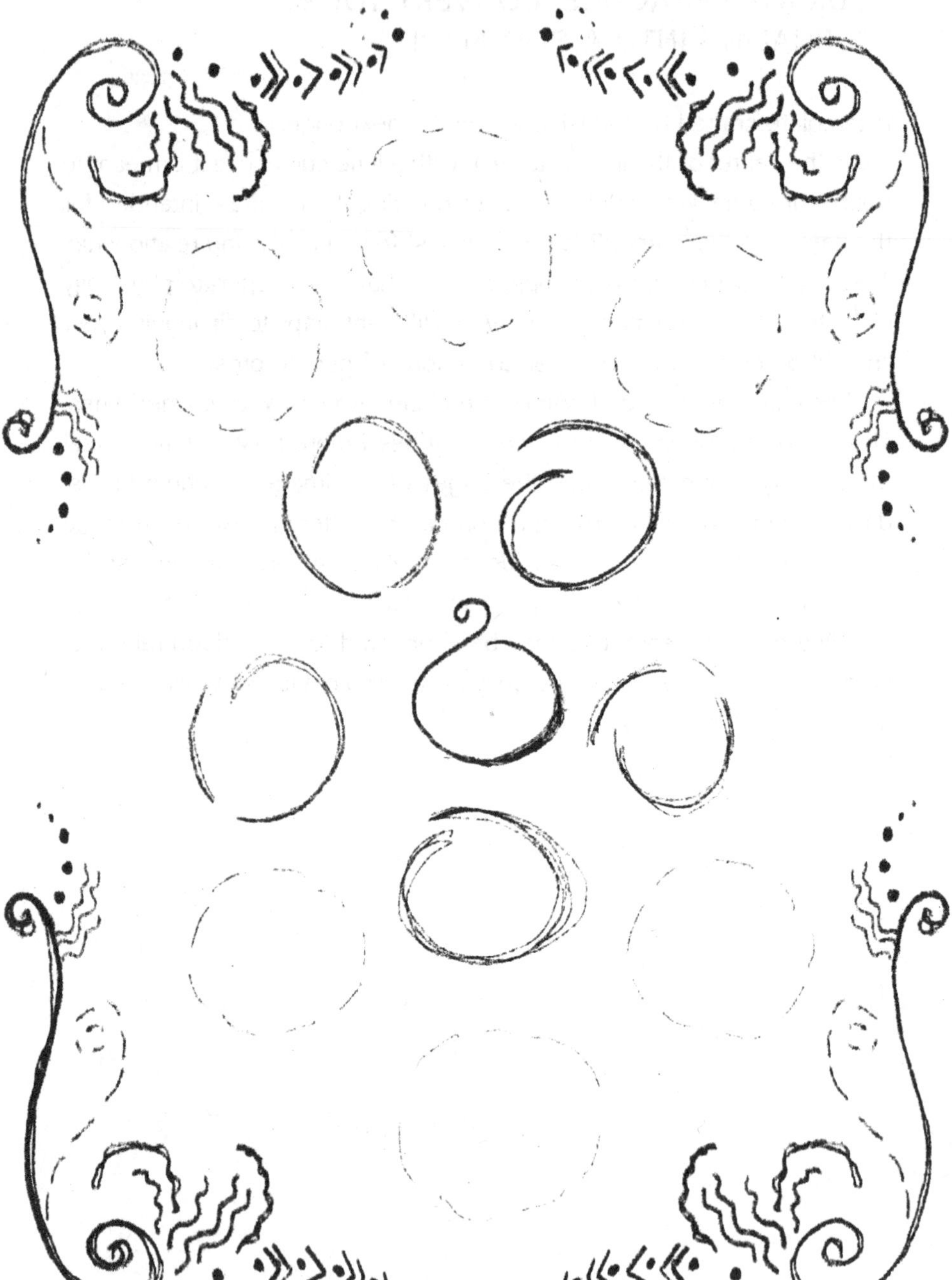

SECTION 3

TAP IN FOR REFLECTION: ACKNOWLEDGE YOUR RITUALS, (RE)ASSESS ASSOCIATIONS WITH SPIRITUALITY

What are some rituals that you engage in regularly for yourself? You can list anything, from the mundane/everyday, like brushing your teeth, to maybe some newer practices you have taken on from this book. You don't need to list every ritual you can think of, just a few that feel important to name.

Once you have populated a small list, revisit the reflection you made on spirituality in Chapter 4 in "Tap in for Reflection: Assess Your Associations with Spirituality." Note anything that has changed (or may be shifting/deepening) in your associations with spiritual practice.

POUR INTO PRACTICE: MAKING TIME FOR "FLOW"

Take a moment to look back at the Pouring into Practice exercises from Sections 1 and 2 (yes, all of them!). We have gradually been encouraging deeper and more extended creative action, from small gestures/doodles, writing exercises, and playlist-building, to larger scale drawing, movement, and poetic (re)construction.

As you review those invitations and your responses to them, is there a particular practice that you can identify where you most felt your body in a state of flow? That is to say, a place where your body felt confident enough in its ability to do what was being asked of you such that the result seemed to pour from you with seemingly minimal effort, or where you may have been so invested in the process that you lost track of the time? Make note of those practices and categorize them in your mind, or on paper, using terms that feel most authentic to you.

As an example, Natasha most easily enters flow state when singing, but small-scale movement is also a place where it can happen. So "singing" and "small-scale movement" would be her terms.

My flow state practices:

Once you've identified those practices, take a look at your schedule for the next week. Where might you make time to dive into a flow sometime in the next seven days? You may have to do some planning here, like thinking about how much time you'll need, where might be the best place to dive in, and what tools you may need to have with you. We will bring you into the practice itself in a later exercise, but just for today, make a plan.

My flow state plan	
What tools will I need?	
When will I be doing this? How much time will I need?	
Where will I be when I'm doing this?	

Lastly, identify someone who you can consider your accountability buddy for this plan. Maybe it's a family member or friend you plan to do the work with, or speak to afterwards about it, or maybe you locate a craft circle or other creative co-work type of environment, where the other people in attendance might serve as the people who can affirm your presence/

commitment to the work. Make sure that some aspect of your community is part of your plan!

My flow state accountability buddy/plan for connecting to community:

POUR INTO PRACTICE: TAKE A MOMENT TO SAY THANK YOU!

Who can you reach out to today to say thank you for their impact on your healing journey? Take a moment to make that connection, whether it's a moment in front of your altar, contacting someone directly, or journaling/scheduling a moment of gratitude for the people who have helped you get where you are today.

Afterwards, let yourself sit with that feeling of gratitude in your body for as long as you feel comfortable. Then, when you're ready, pick up the tools you identified at the end of the last chapter in "Pour into Practice: Making Time for 'Flow'"—we're going right into the practice!

POUR INTO PRACTICE: ENACT YOUR "FLOW STATE PLAN!"

It's time to enter flow!

1. Gather your tools, whether for visual art-making, musicking, writing, movement, or whatever terms you devised in "Pour into Practice: Making Time for 'Flow'" for defining what practices were most "flow-accessible" for you.

2. Set them in front of you (whether literally or in your mind), and take a moment to center yourself and get grounded in your body.

3. When you feel grounded, pick up your tools (again, literally or in your mind), and take another moment to (re)ground yourself, with your tools at the ready.

4. When ready, you are going to engage in a small, repetitive gesture. You can change the speed or the direction of your gesture with each repeat, but the size of the gesture itself should not change.
    a. For visual art-making, this might be a single stroke of your tool, repeated over and over again.
    b. For movement or musicking, you might begin with a small movement, a single note, and develop it into a short pattern of movement or sound that you will repeat.

5. Let yourself explore every possible variation that comes to your mind outside of the size of the gesture itself. Eventually, a state of flow should develop, and when you feel that, *then* you can let go of the size of the gesture and allow it to shift. As that last parameter releases, flow into what emerges from there.

6. When you feel a sense of completion, stop to pause and observe whatever may be happening in your body/mind. If what's happening includes an urge to re-enter the flow, go ahead! You may

pause and resume as many times as feels meaningful, or stop after the first pause.

Journal anything that feels significant in response to this experience. Then, step away from this book, and let what you've experienced marinate.

The work will still be here, and you'll be stronger for the break as well!

Additional space for journaling...

POUR INTO PRACTICE: DEVELOPING A MINI-RITUAL OF CARE

As a child, I (Natasha) attended a Catholic school that was right next to a hospital; in particular, it was right next to the landing for the medical helicopters that would occasionally come in. The sound of whirring chopper blades, to this day, urges me in my sixth-grade teacher's voice to stop whatever I am doing and say a quiet prayer for whoever is inside. In recounting this story to my spouse, he told me of his Mexican grandmother doing something similar—stopping to pray for passing ambulances, a practice I have also taken on, though my "prayers" these days are often no more than a deep breath, because sometimes the moment passes quickly and words are scant. Another place I often stop to take a breath of prayer is any time I pass by any sort of police activity, especially if anyone Black is nearby.

In adopting these practices, no matter how small they may seem, I extend care to myself, or to another person, or a situation, in a ritual way; these are efforts to contribute, however possible, to the highest good of a given moment.

What situations might benefit from you creating similar mini-rituals of care? Your mini-ritual does not have to contain words or any major actions. It can be as simple as: "When I see/experience X, I will take a deep breath."

Whenever you engage in your mini-ritual, make note of any shifts that occur in your body/mind. As you are able, take time to tell someone about what you experienced each time as well. If they feel comfortable, you can invite them to take a breath with you. If this is someone you see or engage with often, maybe this can become a practice that you share.

REFLECTION: RE-MEMBERING LOVE

Take a moment to sit with your body and the decision you made to pick up this book and to embark on this journey with yourself, and with us. We're going to call that choice an act of love. What happens in your body when you do this?

In what other ways do you show love for yourself, and for your people? For the planet?

Who can you talk to about this? Make a point to identify that person and make a plan to share some of what you're reflecting on here before going on with your day.

REFLECTION: RE-MEMBERING YOURSELF THROUGH BEING "WRONG"

How would you describe your relationship with being wrong? Is it something that happens to you often? How accustomed would you say you are to that experience?

Think back to a recent (low stakes, nothing too intense) moment of being wrong. What did you experience in your body the moment you realized that your actions had contributed to what was going on?

Now take a moment to remind your body of the sensation of making something "better" from the first exercise in this book, "Tap in for Reflection: Describe Sensations, Let Memory Support You." Can you feel it? Let yourself deeply remember that feeling.

Now you're going to try and connect the two: that feeling of something getting "better," and the experience of being "wrong." What lives between those two feelings? Maybe this will involve remembering a moment where you made something better after being wrong, or someone helped you to make things better, regardless of who was "wrong." Take a moment to jot down, or maybe even map out, the points of connection from "wrong" to "better" as best you can.

Take breaks if you need to check in with your body and meet its needs before continuing. And don't be afraid to involve other people in this exercise as well, if there's someone you feel the need to consult with for refreshing your memory or taking some other action this experience may motivate you to take.

POUR INTO PRACTICE: MAPPING THE BUILDING BLOCKS OF ACCOUNTABILITY: IDENTITY, NOURISHMENT, BALANCE, AND COMMITMENT

This exercise will be most meaningful when it is completed by more than two people. Bring some of the folks from your (hopefully) growing pod together to do this with you.

For accessibility purposes, the image is briefly described below. The main book also contains a short list of the questions/prompts in text-only form. Below, the questions/prompts are provided with journaling space, for those who'd prefer to engage in this exercise in a linear way. You may also wish to craft your own imagery around these questions, and that is welcome as well!

At the end of the image description and questions/prompts list, an enlarged image-based version can be accessed digitally for sharing and printing so you can lay your papers next to each other after filling it out and make even deeper meaning, as the lines of weaving from side to side and top to bottom should form some interesting links!

Here is the image description: three rectangular patches are laid out vertically over wide bands that weave horizontally across the page. Each patch and band contains prompts and space for writing in responses.

I AM (you can use any descriptive word (adjective) or noun here):

I AM NOT:

Love for myself looks like:

Love for my people looks like:

Love from my people looks like:

This is the kind of (circle one) work/experience/space (or relationship) that nourishes me (this is the place for action words (verbs) or descriptors):

Why? What happens when I am nourished?

How? What are the factors that contribute to my nourishment?

What happens when I am feeling malnourished?

What are the factors that help me balance my nourishment with other folks' needs?

Today I commit to:

My Ancestors remind me:

I welcome:

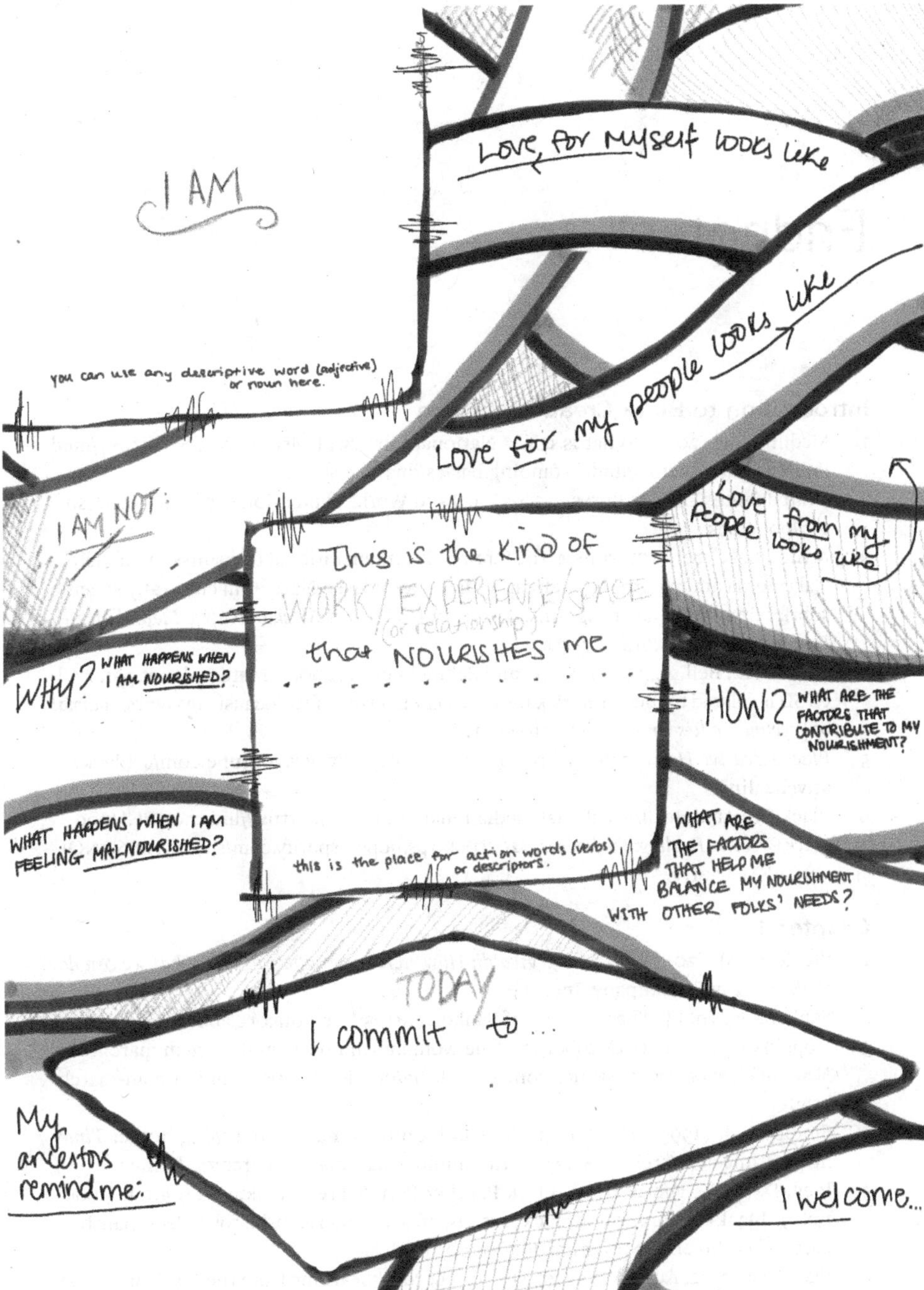

The prompts written in this image are available as a list on page 152 of this book.

Endnotes

Introduction to Black Creative Healing

1 MedlinePlus (2021). What is DNA? National Library of Medicine (US). https://medlineplus.gov/genetics/understanding/basics/dna
2 United States Census Bureau (2025). US and World Population Clock. www.census.gov/popclock
3 Myhra, L. L. (2011). "It runs in the family": Intergenerational transmission of historical trauma among urban American Indians and Alaska Natives in culturally specific sobriety maintenance programs. *American Indian and Alaskan Native Mental Health Research (Online)*, 18(2), 17–40.
4 Yehuda, R., Bell, A., Bierer, L. M., and Schmeidler, J. (2008). Maternal, not paternal, PTSD is related to increased risk for PTSD in offspring of Holocaust survivors. *Journal of Psychiatric Research*, 42(13), 1104–1111.
5 *Black Creative Healing: the Videoblog* (2019). https://www.youtube.com/@blackcreativehealing
6 Black Creative Healing's Social Media Linktree. (2019). https://linktr.ee/BCHpod
7 *Black Creative Healing: the Podcast* (2020). https://open.spotify.com/show/5FsE6ONOIG83xqFMshzzIN

Chapter 1

1 Steele, C. M. (2010). *Whistling Vivaldi: How stereotypes affect us and what we can do*. W.W. Norton & Company, Inc.
2 Sankofa.org (n.d.). The meaning of Sankofa. https://sankofa.org/about
3 Hopkinson, N. (2020, October 17). The women behind the million man march. *The New York Times*. www.nytimes.com/2020/10/17/opinion/women-million-man-march.html
4 Smolowe, J. (1995, October 30). The million man march: Marching home. *Time*. https://time.com/archive/6728084/the-million-man-march-marching-home
5 Pien, D. (2010, February 11). Black Panther Party's Free Breakfast Program (1969–1980). BlackPast.org. www.blackpast.org/african-american-history/black-panther-partys-free-breakfast-program-1969-1980
6 BlackPast (2012, August 12). (1982) Audre Lorde, "Learning from the 60s." BlackPast.org. www.blackpast.org/african-american-history/1982-audre-lorde-learning-60s
7 Shapiro, L. (2022). *The somatic therapy workbook: Stress-relieving exercises for strengthening the mind-body connection and sparking emotional and physical healing*. Ulysses Press.

Chapter 2

1 Yehuda, R., Bell, A., Bierer, L. M., and Schmeidler, J. (2008). Maternal, not paternal, PTSD is related to increased risk for PTSD in offspring of Holocaust survivors. *Journal of Psychiatric Research, 42*(13), 1104–1111.

2 Myhra, L. L. (2011). "It runs in the family": Intergenerational transmission of historical trauma among urban American Indians and Alaska Natives in culturally specific sobriety maintenance programs. *American Indian and Alaskan Native Mental Health Research (Online), 18*(2), 17–40.

3 Alexander, M. (2012). *The new Jim Crow: Mass incarceration in the age of colorblindness.* The New Press.

4 Coker Ross, C. (2024). Slavery and race-based trauma: The impact of historical and intergenerational trauma on health. In N. Kim, C. Coker Ross, M. Fuller, and C. Small (Eds.), *Antiblackness and the Stories of Authentic Allies* (pp. 13–26). Oxford University Press.

5 Coker Ross, C. (2024). Slavery and race-based trauma: The impact of historical and intergenerational trauma on health. In N. Kim, C. Coker Ross, M. Fuller, and C. Small (Eds.), *Antiblackness and the Stories of Authentic Allies* (pp. 13–26). Oxford University Press.

6 DeGruy, J. (2017) *Post traumatic slave syndrome: America's legacy of enduring injury and healing.* Joy DeGruy Publications Inc.

7 Equal Justice Initiative (2017). Lynching in America. https://lynchinginamerica.eji.org

8 Muhammad, K. G. (2010). *The condemnation of Blackness: Race, crime, and the making of modern urban America.* Harvard University Press.

9 Wilkerson, I. (2010). *The warmth of other suns: The epic story of America's great migration.* Vintage Books.

10 Fain, K. (2017, July 5). The devastation of Black Wall Street. https://daily.jstor.org/the-devastation-of-black-wall-street

11 Alexander, M. (2012). *The new Jim Crow: Mass incarceration in the age of colorblindness, revised edition.* The New Press.

12 Diep, W. (2025, February 7). Race conscious admissions and Black students: The past, present, and future. National College Attainment Network. www.ncan.org/news/693186/Race-Conscious-Admissions-and-Black-Students-The-Past-Present-and-Future

13 The Sentencing Project (2024, May 21). Mass incarceration trends. www.sentencingproject.org/reports/mass-incarceration-trends

14 Amihere, D., and Caiola, S. (2022, November 15). Understanding the stop and frisk debate in Philadelphia. WHYY. https://whyy.org/articles/understanding-stop-and-frisk-in-five-charts

15 New York Civil Liberties Union (2025, May 27). Stop-and-frisk data. www.nyclu.org/data/stop-and-frisk-data

16 Schwartz, S. A. (2020). Police brutality and racism in America. *Explore (NY), 16*(5), 280–282.

17 Nurse, A. (2022). *Reparations and anti-black racism: A criminological exploration of the harms of slavery and racialised injustice.* Bristol University Press.

18 Bor, J., Venkataramani, A. S., Williams, D. R., and Tsai, A. C. (2018). Police killings and their spillover effects on the mental health of Black Americans: A population-based, quasi-experimental study. *The Lancet, 392*(10144), 302–310.

19 Abel, M. (2023, September 22). Biases against Black-sounding first names can lead to discrimination in hiring, especially when employers make decisions in a hurry.

The Conversation. https://theconversation.com/biases-against-black-sounding-first-names-can-lead-to-discrimination-in-hiring-especially-when-employers-make-decisions-in-a-hurry-new-research-208423

20 Bouie, J. (May 13, 2015). A tax on Blackness: Racism is still rampant in real estate. *Slate.* https://slate.com/news-and-politics/2015/05/racism-in-real-estate-landlords-redlining-housing-values-and-discrimination.html

21 Diep, W. (2025, February 7). Race conscious admissions and Black students: The past, present, and future. National College Attainment Network. www.ncan.org/news/693186/Race-Conscious-Admissions-and-Black-Students-The-Past-Present-and-Future

22 Bunn, C. (2020, June 23). How LeBron James has become a leading voice for social justice in a racially divided nation. NBC News. www.nbcnews.com/news/nbcblk/how-lebron-james-has-become-leading-voice-social-justice-racially-n1231391

23 Chen, L. (2020, September 15). Dear LeBron James: If you really care about social justice, here's what you should do. *Evie Magazine.* www.eviemagazine.com/post/dear-lebron-james-if-you-really-care-about-social-justice-heres-what-you

24 Menakem, R. (2017). *My grandmother's hands: Racialized trauma and the pathway to mending our hearts and bodies* (p. 8). Central Recovery Press.

25 Williams, D. R., and Williams-Morris, R. (2000). Racism and mental health: The African-American experience. *Ethnicity and Health,* 5(3/4), 243–268.

Chapter 3

1 Saad, L. (2020). *Me and white supremacy: A guided journal* (p. 22). Quercus.

2 Menakem, R. (2017). *My grandmother's hands: Racialized trauma and the pathway to mending our hearts and bodies* (p. 8). Central Recovery Press.

Chapter 4

1 Some, M. P. (1999). *The healing wisdom of Africa.* Tarcher-Putnam.

2 Ferris, W. (2019). The physical aspects of grief. In H. R. Glazer and M. Clark-Foster (Eds.), *Understanding the journey: A lifespan approach to working with grieving people* (pp. 3–16). Charles C. Thomas Publishers.

3 Jegede, A. S. (2002). The Yoruba cultural construction of health and illness (p. 323). *Nordic Journal of African Studies, 11*(3), 322–335.

4 Ayinde, O., Ojagbemi, A., Mankanjuola, V., and Gureje O. (2021). African religions spirituality, and mental health healing practices. In A. Moreira-Almeida, B. Mosquiero, and D. Bhugra (Eds.), *Spirituality and mental health across cultures* (pp. 277–292). Oxford University Press.

5 Ayinde, O., Ojagbemi, A., Mankanjuola, V., and Gureje O. (2021). African religions spirituality, and mental health healing practices. In A. Moreira-Almeida, B. Mosquiero, and D. Bhugra (Eds.), *Spirituality and mental health across cultures* (pp. 277–292). Oxford University Press.

6 Ayinde, O., Ojagbemi, A., Mankanjuola, V., and Gureje O. (2021). African religions spirituality, and mental health healing practices. In A. Moreira-Almeida, B. Mosquiero, and D. Bhugra (Eds.), *Spirituality and mental health across cultures* (pp. 277–292). Oxford University Press.

Chapter 5

1 Little, T. A. (2021). Presentation on spiritual warfare and liberation. Million Artist Movement.

2 Appiah, K. A (2020, October 7). What we can learn from the rise and fall of political blackness. *New York Times*. www.nytimes.com/2020/10/07/opinion/political-blackness-race.html

3 Morrison, T. (1975, May 30). A humanist view [speech transcript]. Portland State University. https://mackenzian.com/wp-content/uploads/2014/07/Transcript_PortlandState_TMorrison.pdf

Chapter 6

1 Braveman, P. and Gottlieb, L. (2014). The social determinants of health: It's time to consider the causes of the causes. *Public Health Reports, 129* (suppl. 2), 19–31.

2 Moonga, N., and Thomas, N. (2025). Orientation to music therapy as a profession. In B., Wheeler, A., Dos Santos, and M. Viega (Eds.), *Music Therapy Handbook* (2nd edition) (pp. 3–18). Buildford Publications.

3 Smith, T. B., Rodríguez, M. D., and Bernal, G. (2011). Culture. In J. C. Norcross (Ed.), *Psychotherapy Relationships that Work* (2nd edition) (pp. 1907–1923). Oxford University Press.

4 Ngwagwa. (2021). Neuroexpansive (TM) thoughts. https://www.instagram.com/p/CYnSGJSrLUz/

5 Linklater, R. (2014). *Decolonizing trauma work: Indigenous stories and strategies*. Fernwood Publishing.

6 Goncalves, J., Lucchetti, G., Menezes, P., and Vallada, H. (2017). Complementary religious and spiritual interventions in physical health and quality of life: A systematic review of randomized controlled clinical trials. *PLoS ONE, 12*(10), e0186539.

7 Thomas, N., Story, K. M., Harman, E., Jacob, S. A., LaMotte, J. E., Kendrick, C., & Robb, S. L. (2025). Music as Supportive Care for Young Children with Sickle Cell Disease and their Parents: A Three-phase Qualitative Exploration into the Cultural Relevance of Active Music Engagement with Black Families. *Global advances in integrative medicine and health*, 14 1–14. https://doi.org/10.1177/27536130251383924

8 U.S. Department of Health and Human Services (n.d.). About the Affordable Care Act: Preventive care. https://www.hhs.gov/healthcare/about-the-aca/index.html

9 Shaw, F., Asomugha, C. N., Conway, P. H., and Rein, A. S. (2014). The Patient Protection and Affordable Care Act: opportunities for prevention and public health. *The Lancet*, 384(9937), 75–82.

10 Bishop, V. (2023, September 8). Time for that tea. *Trinidad Express*. https://trinidadexpress.com/features/local/time-for-that-tea/article_e11ed052-4eb2-11ee-b78a-3763c7b8efaa.html

11 Du, H., Li, X., Lin, D., and Tam, C. C. (2015). Collectivistic orientation, acculturative stress, cultural self-efficacy, and depression: A longitudinal study among Chinese internal migrants. *Community Mental Health Journal, 51*(2), 239–248.

12 Moonga, N., and Thomas, N. (2025). Orientation to music therapy as a profession. In B., Wheeler, A., Dos Santos, and M. Viega (Eds.), *Music Therapy Handbook* (2nd edition) (pp. 3–18). Buildford Publications.

Chapter 7

1 Apter, A. (2013). M. G. Smith on the Isle of Lesbos: Kinship and sexuality in Carriacou. *New West Indian Guide*, 87(3–4), 273–293.

2 Murray, S. O., and Roscoe, W. (2023). *Boy wives and female husbands: Studies in African homosexualities.* SUNY Press.

3 Apter, A. (2013). M. G. Smith on the Isle of Lesbos: Kinship and sexuality in Carriacou. *New West Indian Guide*, 87(3–4), 273–293.

4 Thomas, N., and Forinash, M. (2024). Queering research. In C. Lee, (Ed.), *Oxford Handbook of Queer and Trans Music Therapy* (pp.483–502). Oxford University Press.

5 Documenting Queerness (n.d.). YouTube Channel. www.youtube.com/@Documenting_Queerness

6 Mingus, M. (2016). Pods and pod mapping worksheet. Bay Area Transformative Justice. https://batjc.org/files/Pods-Pod-Mapping-Worksheet.pdf

Chapter 8

1 Some, M. P. (1999). *The healing wisdom of Africa.* Tarcher-Putnam.

2 Some, M. P. (1999). *The healing wisdom of Africa.* Tarcher-Putnam. p. 190.

3 Csikszentmihalyi, M. (2008). Flow, the secret to happiness. TED Talk. www.youtube.com/watch?v=fXIeFJCqsPs

Chapter 9

1 Monte, L. M. and Perez-Lopez, D. J. (2021, July 21). COVID-19 pandemic hit Black households harder than white households, even when pre-pandemic socio-economic disparities are taken into account. www.census.gov/library/stories/2021/07/how-pandemic-affected-black-and-white-households.html

2 Vasquez Reyes M. (2020). The disproportional impact of COVID-19 on African Americans. *Health and Human Rights*, 22(2), 299–307.

3 Laskshmi Piepzna-Samarashina, L. (2018). *Carework: Dreaming disability justice.* Arsenal Pulp Press.

4 Friedman, C. (2022). COVID-19 infection differences among people with disabilities. *Dialogues in Health*, 1, 100083.

5 Wendel, C. L., Gray, R. C., Goddard, K., and Hall, J. P. (2024). Navigating new normals: The influence of COVID-19 policies on community access and well-being of people with mobility disabilities in everyday life. *Frontiers in Public Health*, 12, 1401777.

Chapter 10

1 hooks, b. (2001). *Salvation: Black people and love.* Harper Collins.

2 hooks, b. (2001). *Salvation: Black people and love.* Harper Collins. p. 4.

3 hooks, b. (2001). *Salvation: Black people and love.* Harper Collins. p. xxiv.

4 Some, S. (2004). *Women's wisdom from the heart of Africa.* (Audiobook.) Sounds True.

5 Garina, D. (n.d.). Centered Accountability Course. https://accountabilitymapping.com

6 Creative Interventions (2021). *Creative Interventions Toolkit.* AK Press.

RAISING READERS

Books Build Bright Futures

Dear Reader,

We'd love your attention for one more page to tell you about the crisis in children's reading, and what we can all do.

Studies have shown that reading for fun is the **single biggest predictor of a child's future life chances** – more than family circumstance, parents' educational background or income. It improves academic results, mental health, wealth, communication skills, ambition and happiness.[1]

The number of children reading for fun is in rapid decline. Young people have a lot of competition for their time. In 2024, 1 in 10 children and young people in the UK aged 5 to 18 did not own a single book at home.[2]

Hachette works extensively with schools, libraries and literacy charities, but here are some ways we can all raise more readers:

- Reading to children for just 10 minutes a day makes a difference
- Don't give up if children aren't regular readers – there will be books for them!
- Visit bookshops and libraries to get recommendations
- Encourage them to listen to audiobooks
- Support school libraries
- Give books as gifts

There's a lot more information about how to encourage children to read on our website: **www.RaisingReaders.co.uk**

Thank you for reading.

hachette UK

---

1 OECD, '21st-Century Readers: Developing Literacy Skills in a Digital World', 2021, https://www.oecd.org/en/publications/21st-century-readers_a83d84cb-en.html

2 National Literacy Trust, 'Book Ownership in 2024', November 2024, https://literacytrust.org.uk/research-services/research-reports/book-ownership-in-2024